The Intermittent Fasting
16/8 Lifestyle

&

The Keto Lifestyle
-2 In 1-

Why Combining Intermittent Fasting With The Ketogenic Diet Is The Best Way For Rapid Weight Loss

By

Jasmine Carter

Table of Contents

The Intermittent Fasting 16/8 Lifestyle

Introduction 8

The Power of Intermittent Fasting 9
What is Fasting? Intermittently? 9

The Protocol.. 14
Preparing for a Lifestyle Change 14
Frequently Asked Questions for Beginners 19
10-Day Intermittent Fasting Routine 23

Changing it Up 36
How to Turn Any Diet into the 16:8 Method............... 36

The Intermittent Fasting Lifestyle..................... 38
Monitor & Assess Progress........................... 38
Hacks to Success...................................... 39
Setbacks... 44
The Lifestyle Change and Daily Routine.................... 49

Conclusion... 52

References 54

The Keto Lifestyle

Introduction 57

Chapter 1-Knowing Deeper the Ketogenic Diet 60
Program Principles & Core Concept 61
Attaining Optimal Ketosis = A-OK! 62
Ketogenesis/Ketosis Macronutrient Model: Ideal
Implementation of the Correct Caloric Configuration
Consumption 64
Keystone Labels for Ketone Levels: Knowing the
Kismets of Ketosis.. 65

Chapter 2-Reaping the Regimen's Remarkable Rewards 68

Chapter 3- Starting & Sticking to the Program's Proper Performances 72
Regimen's Requirements & Regulations 73
Rationalizing Rated Ratios 74

Chapter 4-Grocery Guide 76
Inclusive Items for Constant Consumption
(Recommended & Restricted Rations) 77

Abbreviations 78

Chapter 5-Bountiful Breakfasts 79
1-Choco Chip Whey Waffles 79
2-Coco Cinnamon-Packed Pancakes 80
3-Magdalena Muffins with Tart Tomatoes 81
4-Spinach Shoots Mediterranean Medley 82
5-Romantic Raspberry Power Pancake 83
6-Spinach Sausage Feta Frittata 84
7-Mayonnaise Mixed with Energy Egg 86
8-Avocados atop Toasted Tartiné 87
9-Fish Fillet & Perky Potato Cheese Combo 88
10-Cream Cheese Protein Pancake 89
11-Veggie Variety with Peanut Paste 90
12-Avocado Aliment with Egg Element 92
13-Pumpkin Pancakes 93
14-Whole-Wheat Plain Pancakes 95
15-Blueberries Breakfast Bowl 96
16-Feta-Filled Tomato-Topped Oldie Omelet 97
17-Ave Avocado Super Smoothie 98
18-Hearty Hodgepodge 99
19-Chocolate Chia Plain Pudding 100
20-Seasoned Sardines with Sunny Side 101

Chapter 6-Luscious Lunch 102
1-Pulled Pepper-Lemon Loins 102
2-Shrimps & Spinach Spaghetti 104
3-Single Skillet Seafood-Filled Frittata 105

4-Poultry Pâté & Creamy Crackers 107
5-Chickpeas Carrots Curry 108
6-Baked Broccoli in Olive Oil..................................... 109
7-Bunless Bacon Burger... 110
8-Smoky Sage Sausage.. 111
9-Steamed Salmon & Salad Bento Box 112
10-Stuffed Spaghetti Squash..................................... 114
11-Prawn Pasta.. 116
12- Tasty Tofu Carrots &Cauliflower Cereal 118
13-Stuffed Straw Mushroom Mobcap 120
14-Crispy Chicken Packed in Pandan 122
15-Chicken Curry Masala Mix 123
16-Milano Meatballs with Tangy Tomato................... 124
17-Aubergine À la Lasagna Lunch............................. 126
18-Beef Broccoli with Sesame Sauce........................ 128
19- Sautéed Sirloin Steak in Sour Sauce 130
20-Flaky Fillets with Garden Greens......................... 132

Chapter 7-Dinner Delights............................... 134
1-Pizza Pie with Cheesy Cauliflower Crust.............. 134
2-Roasted Rib-eye Skillet Steak 136
3-À la Spaghetti with Asian Sauce 137
4-Shirataki & Soy Sprouts Pad Thai with Peanut
Tidbits 138
5-Charred Chicken with Squash Seed Sauce........... 140
6-Therapeutic Turmeric & Shirataki Soup................. 142
7-Fresh Fettuccine with Pumpkin Pesto 143
8- Cheddar Chicken Casserole 145
9-Zesty Zucchini Pseudo Pasta & Sweet Spanish
Onions Overload 146
10-Soba & Spinach Sprouts....................................... 147
11-Chickpeas & Carrot Consommé 149
12-Chicken Cauliflower Curry..................................... 151
13-Cheesy Cauliflower Mac Munchies 153
14-Sugar Snap Pea Pods with Coco Crunch............ 154
15-Spicy & Smoky Spinach-Set Fish Fillets 155
16-Spicy Shrimps & Sweet Shishito 157
17-Spaghetti-Styled Zesty Zucchini with Guacamole
Garnish 158

18-Grain-less Gnocchi in Melted Mozzarella 160
19-Cauliflower Chao Fan Fried with Pork Pastiche . 161
20-All-Avocado Stuffed with Spicy Beef Bits 163

Chapter 8-Satisfying Snacks 164
1-Coconut Candy.. 164
2-Mozzarella Mound Munchies 165
3-Philadelphia Potato Praline 166
4-Tasty Turkey Cheese Cylinders 167
5-Fried Flaxseed Tortilla Treat.................................. 168
6-Power-Packed Butter Balls..................................... 169
7-Choco Coco Cups 170
8-Corndog Clumps 171
9-Kingly Kale Crispy Chips 173
10-Ambrosial Avocado Puree Pudding 174

Chapter 9-Delectable Desserts......................... 175
1-Cool Cucumber Sushi with Sriracha Sauce 175
2-Coco Crack Bake-less Biscuit Bars........................ 177
3-Chocolate-Coated Sweet Strawberries 178
4-Matcha Muffins with Choco-Coco Coating............ 179
5-Cinnamon Cup Cake... 180
6-Choco 'Cado Twin Truffles 182
7-Butter Ball Bombs.. 183
8-Choco Coco Cookies... 184
9-Carrot Compact Cake 185
10-Chilled Cream 186
Cooking Calibrations & Conversion Charts 187

Chapter 10-Daily Dietary Planning Programs. 190
Calorie Consumption Calculation 190
7-Day Dietary Planning Program (1,500 Calorie
Consumption) 192
7-Day Dietary Planning Program (1,750 Calorie
Consumption) 200
7- Day Dietary Planning Program (2,000 Calorie
Consumption) 207

Conclusion 214

References 217

Disclaimer **219**

The Intermittent Fasting 16/8 Lifestyle

How I Lost 10 Lbs. In A Month While
Still Eating All My Favorite Foods

By

Jasmine Carter

Introduction

Most people would agree that dieting is stressful, there are too many diet options, and most diets are not sustainable, leaving them to believe losing or maintaining weight is impossible. What if I told you I knew a way for you to successfully eat the meals that you desire and eat your absolute favorite foods, when you wanted too, in the easiest and fastest way, and still lose weight and/or maintain weight depending on your meal choices? Would you be interested? Ok, great. In this book, you will learn how to change your eating habits to accommodate a new lifestyle to allow you to lose weight and/or maintain weight loss. This new habit and lifestyle change is called Intermittent Fasting.

Some advantages of this lifestyle are as follows: there is no food group that must be excluded, you can select your meals and when to eat, there are no types of purchases that must be made, you will see a spike in your energy level, and more.

It was only 483 days ago that I and my wife was considered obese and were unable to conceive. Together and individually, we had tried many of the available options to include: Adkins Diet, Keto Diet, Low Carb Diet, No Sugar Diet, No Meat Diet, Vegan Diet, Weight Watchers, Raw Food Diet, and more. Because of this new lifestyle change, together we successfully lost over 160 lbs. and have maintained the weight loss for over a year and are now proud parents of a baby boy. This lifestyle change made it easy for us to adapt, and as a bonus of losing and maintaining this weight loss, we were able to naturally conceive.

By continuing to read this book, you will have all the tools to lose weight and maintain that weight loss in one place. This book explains the lifestyle change, how it works, and the science behind how it works. It also documents details on how to set up your new lifestyle, key information to know before starting, best tips for beginners, an actual daily protocol, how to monitor your progress, how to deal with setbacks, and much more! These and more details have proven a success; this book will ensure a lifestyle change and give you complete weight management. Start today, you can lose 10 pounds in the first week and keep it off forever!

The Power of Intermittent Fasting

What is Fasting? Intermittently?

Fasting is a choice to abstain from eating and/or drinking for a period. Intermittent Fasting is an eating lifestyle, in which you only eat during a specific feeding window, and not consume calories during your fasting window. A feeding window is a time in which you have decided to intake calories. A fasting window is a time in which you have decided NOT to consume calories.

Intermittent Fasting, or "IF", is the process of choosing a feeding window and a fasting window that equals 24 hours in your day. This is a lifestyle choice that does not rely on food restrictions like other types of diet tactics. Intermittent Fasting is popular today because it is now associated with weight management and weight loss and offers many benefits without much effort besides deciding and committing to the feeding and fasting windows that you have chosen. [1] There are multiple methods in which people choose to fast, sometimes by hours, sometimes by days, sometimes by meals. The emphasis here will be on the basic feeding/fasting windows in a daily hourly method.

Intermittent Fasting 16:8 Method

The Intermittent Fasting 16:8 Method is when you fast 16 hours out of the day, and only eat during a total of 8 hours a day. The fasting window is a total of 16 hours a day; Your fasting window will mostly be during the time you are sleeping. During your fasting window, you will NOT consume ANY calories at all. Not eating when your mind and body are accustomed to eating will be difficult, but the challenge is mind over matter, and you matter, so you will succeed. Choose a time to start and stop your feeding window, when the feeding window stops, the fasting window starts, and when the fasting window stops, the feeding window starts, and so on.

The Benefits & Why the 16:8 Method

Intermittent Fasting is not complicated, and it does not have to affect the way you live your daily life. This lifestyle will compliment your current life and not work against it. You will still be able to enjoy dinner with your family, happy hour with your friends, and a drink after dinner if you want. Living this lifestyle, there is no predetermined time that must be used as the feeding and/or fasting window, this is your choice; the fasting and feeding times can be set according to your current personal schedule.

With the other diets, you must exclude carbs, sugars, meats, alcohol, social outings, your wants, flavors, fats, and/or more, but with IF you DO NOT have to exclude a food group if you do not choose to. Other diet tactics, take too much mental space to keep up; there are way too many food restrictions and rules. With the 16:8 method, some people even consume fewer calories, and sometimes fewer meals, than they plan to because you are only eating during your 8-hour feeding window and you are accustomed to eating more or longer hours in a day.

With this method, you do not have to eat breakfast, but you can eat breakfast if you want at whatever time you choose. Breakfast is considered the first meal of the day and has always been recognized as the most important meal of the day, you can still have this meal, it may just be at a different time than the average person considers breakfast time. Your breakfast, lunch, and dinner times may be at average times if you want or they can be non-traditional times, this is again your choice when living an IF lifestyle. You do not have to stop eating by 6pm, 7pm, or 8pm; You stop eating when your feeding window is over, based on the time you have chosen.

There are no supplements or disgusting shakes or drinks that you are required to ingest at certain times a day every day. There are no books or journals or apps you must purchase or carry around with you to have to keep track of your meals, or the calories, or macros, or carbs, etc. You are not required to increase your spending in any way to start or maintain an IF lifestyle, which is the ultimate advantage of living this lifestyle. Any person with any income with any type of career and schedule can use the 16:8 method of intermittent fasting.

Some people struggle with food cravings, emotional eating habits, food addictions and triggers, binge eating, food obsessiveness, and more. These habits could be physiological or psychological, depends on the individual. Physiological eating habits are healthier and the end goal. Psychological eating habits are displayed in a person when they have eaten and are physically full, there is no actual physical hunger pains or needs at that time, but they still eat more for innumerable reasons in their head. The first week or so of this lifestyle change to Intermittent Fasting could help people recognize the differences between physical hunger and psychological hunger.

Leangains Method

The 16:8 Method is also known as the Leangains Method, coined by Martin Berkhan. This is a high protein eating lifestyle, which is focused on carb, fat, and protein ratio, these are called your macronutrients. The Leangains Method or protocol also promotes exercise heavily.

On workout days, the largest meal of the day should be the post-workout meal. It consists of high carbs, moderate proteins, and low fat. On non-work out days, the largest meal should be the first meal of the day, and because there is no workout that day the calorie intake should be less, the fat intake should be higher, along with fibrous veggies, meat, and fruit as the components of this meal, there should be little to no carb intake. Dinner, the last meal of each day, should consist of slow digesting protein options like eggs, fish, nut butter, dairy, and more. These types of food before bed keeps the body nourished during sleep and the fasted state. [10]

How does IF Work?

This type of fasting is NOT all hype with no context; there is science behind the efficacy of intermittent fasting on human health. There are many health benefits, in addition to weight loss and/or weight management, as discussed previously. Blood pressure, triglycerides, fat mass, blood glucose, LDL cholesterol, and blood sugars all improve, as intermittent fasting becomes more and more familiar within your body system. [2]

Intermittent fasting has been associated with diabetes prevention and has resulted in the reprieve of pre-diabetic symptoms. Sugar is what our cells use for energy. If our cells don't use it for energy, the sugar is stored as fat within our fat cells. Sugar can only enter our cells with insulin. Insulin is what brings sugar into our fat cells and keeps it there. Intermittent Fasting lowers insulin levels, which prevents our fat cells from holding on to stored sugar in our bodies, which inevitably, if not released, causes a decrease in energy. The longer a person fasts, the more fat cells your body will burn for fuel instead of storing as body fat, which will result in increased energy. [12]

Intermittent fasting also significantly improves insulin sensitivity. Insulin sensitivity describes how sensitive the body is to the effects of insulin; having a good sensitivity to insulin is a sign of good health. Intermittent Fasting drops your insulin levels, which alters your body's demand for insulin in a good way, it also resets your insulin sensitivity.[3] Of lately, intermittent fasting has been associated with preserving memory and learning functionality; once your body starts using its fat stores for energy, ketones are then used, which is what protects the neurons for memory and learning functions.[4,15]

Like with exercise, Intermittent fasting puts your bodies cells under mild stress. A physiological benefit of intermittent fasting is that your body learns to cope with this stress and fight back, hence resist disease more and more as your body learns to cope. This fasting is associated with making your bodies overall health stronger. Intermittent Fasting is reportedly been associated with an influence on metabolic regulations, this includes circadian rhythm, gut microbes, and modifiable lifestyle behaviors.

Humans have evolved to perform most physiological processes at optimal times; certain activities are optimally done during the day hours and others, like sleep, are done at night, this is what most people call natural. A circadian rhythm is the regular recurrence of life activities in a 24-hour cycle. Consuming food outside of the normal feed phase, which is during the night hours when people should be sleep, resets some circadian rhythms and disrupts energy balance; hence a major effect on a persons metabolism. Any fasting that encourages NOT eating during the night hours allowing the body to burn fatter, synchronizes food intake with the optimal times to eat. [2, 16]

Having an intermittent fasting lifestyle seems to have a positive impact on gut microbiota. Gut microbiota is a complex community of microorganisms that live in your digestive tract. This positivity also goes along with the circadian rhythms. Gastric emptying and blood flow function optimally during the daytime rather than at night, so disturbing circadian may negatively affect gastrointestinal functions and ultimately impair metabolism and health.[3]

Intermittent fasting has improved self-reported sleep satisfaction. Night time eating has been associated with sleep deprivation and insomnia, which can have negative effects on insulin resistance. Insulin resistance increases the risk of Diabetes and other cardiovascular diseases. The increased effects of prolonged nightly fasting can prevent Diabetes, other cardiovascular diseases, negative insulin resistance, insomnia, and/or sleep deprivation. [1]

The Protocol

Preparing for a Lifestyle Change

How to Start (Setting up Fasting and Feeding Times)

To get started all you need is a good idea of your daily routine schedule, on average, as each day is not created equal for sure. Think back and jot down the time frame in which you think you do most of your eating on an average day. Next, jot down the time in which you think you get the most sleep. Lastly, jot down other important time frames that are important to your average daily routine. Some important time frames I jotted down and considered initially were happy hours with my spouse and friends, and family dinner time, in which we eat dinner together each day.

I considered that on average, my eating times ranged from 10:00 AM to about 8:00 PM on weekdays and from 12:00 PM to midnight on the weekends, as I have a great social life. With terrible sleeping habits, I was sleeping around midnight, waking up at 8:00 AM at the latest on weekdays and from 2:00 AM to 12:00 PM on weekends.

Review your notes and decide on the best 8 hours out of your day to be considered your feeding window. With this schedule, I would say a good starting feeding window would be 12:00 PM to 8:00 PM daily. With this feeding window, the fasting window would automatically be daily starting at 8:00 PM and fast until 12:00 PM. Some people consume 3 meals during this 8-hour window, but I found that to be impossible for me, so I consume 2 moderate portioned sized meals and eat snacks at other times during the feeding window. You can decide to eat how many meals and snacks you want while intermittent fasting, but decide and be consistent.

Meal Planning

Meal planning, also known as meal prep, is NOT required to be successful with intermittent fasting, however, it does a good job of preparing you for even more success with your feeding window. Meal prep is preparing some or all meals/snacks in advance to have on hand when needed. Meal prep saves you time, so you aren't preparing meals/snacks each day and it takes away the thought process of what you will eat during your feeding windows daily. By meal prepping, there is less room for failure, especially for beginners. With meal planning comes the bonus of preparing healthier options to eat during your feeding window, instead of choosing quickly processed and prepacked options because it's convenient.

For me there are many steps to Meal Planning. Meal Planning consists of creating full meals (this includes recipes), creating all-inclusive grocery lists, reviewing your own kitchen to see what you already have and what you need, then altering your grocery list, and finally going grocery shopping.

Creating meals takes creativity. With the world wide web, there are plenty of recipes and meals ideas for available options. Being creative means not always eating the same thing day in and day out. Change up your breakfast options, lunch options, dinner options, and snacks. Season the food differently. Cook a different cut of the beef. Garnish it differently. Make it a soup or salad instead of a casserole. Make vegetables a snack in some way. Find ways to increase your protein intake. Add more green leaves to your protein shakes and/or more vegetables or fruits. Decide on 2-3 lunch and dinner options, and 2-3 snack options.

Once you have decided on what meals you have created and the recipes, you will need to search through your kitchen cabinets, freezer, pantry, and refrigerator to see what you have already have and don't need to purchase when you go food shopping. This includes everything, meats, sides, fresh vegetables, fresh fruit, drinks, snack options, spices, herbs, oils, breads, wraps, and more. Revise your grocery shopping list to include what you need.

Proceed to go to the grocery stores and pick up the items on your list. In preparation for meal prep. Meal prep is taking all of your groceries and cutting up everything that needs to be cut up, washing everything that needs to be washed, marinating everything that needs to be marinated, seasoning everything that needs to be seasoned, baking everything that needs to be backed, cooking everything that needs to be cooked, measure everything that needs to be measured to the appropriate portion, and packing it all in individual meal Tupperware containers to easily grab and go when needed. Although highly recommended, meal planning and prep, is NOT required for intermittent fasting.

Portion Control, Food Labels, & Measurements

Portion control is NOT necessarily required when intermittent fasting, however, because you are not restricting any food groups and you can technically eat what you want during your feeding window, portion control becomes even more important than meal prep, but could also work in speeding up the weight loss when treated equally. Portion control does not mean you have to eat tiny portions of everything. Portion control is the serving size on the label or the amount that is generally served. To best practice portion control when your meal prep, measure your foods and package them into the containers before storing them away for later meals. Another tip to use, to ensure you are eating proportionately, is to drink a glass of water to ensure you are hungry and not just thirsty and to ensure you do not overeat.

Food Labels displays the nutrient content/nutritional facts, calories, and serving sizes for packaged foods. Reading food labels will ensure you are not eating too much at one time, this is fundamentally portion control at its best. The first things to review is the serving size. Serving size is the portion size that is generally served at once. The calorie count displays how many calories are in one serving. Food labels also include the total fats, cholesterol, sodium, and total carbohydrates per serving size. Additionally, the % daily value displays how much this serving will count towards your daily intake, try not to go over 100% in any category. Reading and understanding food labels are NOT required to be successful while intermittent fasting, but this could enhance results.

Counting net carbs is another big topic of discussion that people tend to gravitate too. To count net carbs, subtract the dietary fiber from the total carbohydrates count, this equals net carbs. Counting net carbs only is an acceptable way to eat and meal plan, BUT counting net carbs is not required to intermittent fast. Counting net carbs and calories are NOT required for intermittent fasting. [17]

Measuring foods is NOT necessarily required when intermittent fasting, but it ensures you are not eating too much of whatever you choose to eat. Use smaller containers to ensure you are eating a good amount of food to be full, but not stuffed. Never eat from the package that the snack came in, and limit distractions while you eat, as people usually overeat while doing activities, such as watching television. Measuring food is important for portion control, but not required for intermittent fasting.

Choose Food Options Wisely/Balanced Options

When following an intermittent fasting lifestyle, you are not restricted from any food group and you can choose your own meal options, BUT food choices are still (as always) important. It is important to have good nutrition that emphasizes a diet that provides a complete source of minerals, vitamins, and nutrients for the healthiest functioning body.

A diet is considered the sum of all foods eaten, but it refers to the use of specific intake of nutrition. Any healthy diet should include whole and unprocessed foods over processed and/or liquid foods to include plenty of fruits and vegetables, lean proteins, some fats and oils, and grains; this would be considered a balanced meal, these are also called energy-dense foods. Energy-dense foods are high in fiber and helps to retain natural water. [14]

When fasting, try to eat more non-starchy vegetables and lean proteins. Choose foods that are whole grain and stay away from refined grains and flours. Fruit is going to be the best option to try to curb the still existing sweet tooth, especially for beginners. Choose a non-dairy over dairy and eat fats and oils in moderation and choose the healthiest forms of fats and oils.

Fresh fruits and vegetables are favored over frozen and canned, but any vegetable is better than no vegetables at all. Choose lean cuts of protein and to increase your protein intake add vegetarian sources, like beans and soy products. Try almond, soy, or cashew non-dairy options to limit your dairy intake, as dairy is one of the world's leading allergens. Other leading allergens include eggs, peanuts, and shellfish. [1] Make carbs toppers instead of the base of your meals. When buying pasta, bread, crackers, and more always look for whole grain listed as the first ingredient on the nutrition label. Eat half of an avocado at least once a day to increase your healthy fat intake.

According to the USDA, there are 5 principle guidelines to follow to satisfy your dietary needs. Follow a healthy eating pattern across your entire lifespan, a lot of people are not following this first guideline. An eating pattern is your liquids and foods intake and your routine way of eating. Following this first guideline ensures nutrient adequacy, healthy body systems, and lower risks to chronic disease invasions of your body. The second and fourth guideline is to focus on the amount of food and liquids you consume and to be focused on eating nutrient-dense foods from all the major food groups and how to shift from bad choices to good choices. The decisions you make are most important. You are the important link that makes the difference, you are in control of ensuring you are meeting these guidelines. Meeting these guidelines is the responsibility of all people.

The third guideline is to limit the number of calories that do not come from nutrient-dense foods, such as added sugars, high sodium, and trans and saturated fats. According to the USDA, healthy eating meals consist of a whole fruit, fresh vegetables, dairy, protein, whole grains, and oils. The fifth guideline is teaching you how to share your knowledge with others; it states that support is necessary for change for everyone and that it is all our jobs to support healthy eating habits. [1]

Physical Activity

Like meal planning, measuring foods, reading food labels, and portion control, exercise is NOT required, but beneficial to your overall results while intermittent fasting. The American Heart Association recommends some form of physical activity for at least 30 minutes daily. [13]

Create a workout schedule. Make a leg day, an arms day, cardio day, total body weight day, and more. A schedule starts to make you more consistent and accountable. On days when you feel unmotivated to do one you have the other. If you are already exercise, intermittent fasting can only improve your results. The combination of intermittent fasting and exercise maximizes weight loss and/or weight maintenance.

Mindset

The biggest barrier, if any, will be your mindset. The barrier will be the already set attitudes and assumptions you have in your head specifically as it relates to the relationship you have with food and eating food. Think mind over matter, and you matter the most to yourself, so take better care of yourself. To sustain following an intermittent lifestyle, you will need to erase or ignore all prior assumptions or attitudes related to diets/lifestyle changes, losing weight, current food habits, current eating schedules, change in general, and more. Once started, try to make optimal choices for you and be disciplined in being consistent in carrying plans throughout. To be successful you will need to think and act differently for optimal results.

Surviving Longer While Hungry

Hunger is feeling uncomfortable and/or being weak due to a lack of food. Hunger can be physical, but it can also just be a desire or want rather than a need right at that moment. The body sometimes responds as if its hunger, but sometimes we are thirsty and are yearning for liquids and not food, therefore your water intake is imperative to your success in extending to longer fasting windows.

To habituate longer fasting windows and/or to resist food during your fasting window to make it to the feeding window, staying productive is vital. Stay busy by any means necessary. It is a great idea to exercise during this time or stay busy with your professional or personal work. Being lazy and feeling bored are false indicators to your body that you may be hungry when really you are just in a slump or bored. The more you think about food the weaker your body thinks your mind is and eventually this will be your takedown.

Frequently Asked Questions for Beginners

Most types of changes come with a lot of questions, intermittent fasting is no different. Here are some frequently asked questions from beginners: How should I schedule my feeding and fasting times if I work overnight or long shifts? Schedule your feeding and fasting window according to your own time, which means your feeding window would be more so evenings and overnight and the fasting more of the daytime when you are sleeping.

Can I have coffee? Yes, you can have black coffee, water, and plain steeped tea.

Can I add cream/sugar/milk in my coffee? The goal of fasting is to not add calories, so the answer is no, you should not add anything to your coffee. However, I have heard of cases in which intermittent fasters add less than 50 calories to their coffee and they have claimed to still be successful with intermittent fasting; I have heard that it does not affect their fasted state, but keep in mind all individuals are not created equal. I would not recommend adding anything to your coffee, but if adding something to your coffee still makes this a good change for the goal you have for yourself then give it a try.

Does intermittent fasting work well with veganism, paleo, keto, vegetarianism, or any other styles of eating? Yes, the beauty of intermittent fasting is that it can be combined with any style of eating unless otherwise directed by a medical professional. You can turn your style of eating into the 16:8 method with ease, as this change does not restrict or state the style/types of food you eat, it is specifically based on the timing of your eating.

Is there an alternative to the 16:8 method if I cannot initially fast 16 hours and want to work my way up to 16? Yes, especially for women, it is recommended that if women cannot or are not willing to do a 16 hour fast, they can start with a 14-hour fasting window and 10-hour feeding window. This is recommended for women, but men can start here if needed. Once the 14 hours is mastered, you can then work your way up to the 16:8 method.

Can I have a cheat meal? You can technically eat what you want when intermittent fasting, there are no food group restrictions. There is no cheat meal to have, unless you have decided that you have put yourself on some type of restrictive meals/foods to not indulge in, if so, then yes, but I recommend to always eat in moderation.

What are some healthy snack foods to eat on the go during my feeding window? Pepperoni slices, fruit, veggie tray, Skinny Pop popcorn individual bags (unless you will always measure the servings before consuming), turkey/beef jerky, individual peanut butter cups, whole grain cereal, almond milk, eggs, rice cakes, nuts (individual bags), hummus, and more.

I am too hungry during my fasting window, what should I do? Be patient and wait for your body to adapt to this change. This may take some time, for some it occurs fast, for others it may take a week or so, but this depends on how you were eating before you began this lifestyle. According to Collier in 2013, your body is still adjusting to how it was functioning before and is fighting you to get back to that way, as most people were eating more frequently and maybe even more meals or snacks during the day. Eventually, you will not feel this way. Eventually, you will adapt to your feeding and fasting windows and the urge to eat or the thought of starving will get easier and easier until it goes away. [11]

Why am I not losing fat faster, like other people are? It is more than likely a combination of not eating the appropriate portions when you are eating and/or not preparing to eat the right food choices. Although fat and weight loss can still happen, its more frequent and visible when the appropriate food choices and portions are selected and prepared.

How can I stay full longer? Eat more fiber and drink more water, stay hydrated.

Do I have to eat low carb? No, you can eat what you want during your feeding window. I recommend eating proportionately and choosing the healthier food options. Instead of white bread choose whole grain bread. Instead of white rice choose brown rice. Instead of anything with high fructose corn syrup, scratch it off, instead of canned fruit, eat fresh fruit.

Should I exercise in the fasted state? You can, but it is not required. It is also not recommended on heavy lifting days.

What if I am on medications and must eat with my morning medications? In this case, you would need to make your feeding window begin at whatever time you take your meds. I would recommend taking your meds as late as you can in the mornings but do get authorization of your plan from a medical professional.

Should I discuss this with my medical professional before beginning the change? Yes, you should always discuss diet changes with a medical professional before you begin.

Frequent Mistakes

People have failed due to the following frequent mistakes. Don't be one of these people, be knowledgeable and plan and think ahead.

One of the biggest mistakes beginners make is not finishing this book to the end and not taking this information seriously; basically, starting too soon, before you are prepared to start. While reading this book, it's a good idea to take notes, and jot down an individual plan while reading and sometimes doing further research during your reading. It wouldn't hurt to even read this book twice, especially if this is your first exposure to fasting, specifically intermittent fasting.

Another mistake that is made, not only with intermittent fasting but with any and most diet plans or lifestyle eating changes, is when people try to implement too many changes at once. It is not a good idea to try to become vegan and implement intermittent fasting at the same time. It is not a good idea to start working out with a trainer 4 days a week and implement intermittent fasting. It is not a good idea to start a new job with varying schedules and implement intermittent fasting at the same time. It is not a good idea to start a new medication, a new workout plan, and intermittent fasting at the same time. Not to say this is impossible, it is, but on average these are too many changes at once for a beginner.

Most of us have been taught to eat 3 good sized meals a day, breakfast, lunch, and dinner (which includes dessert) and to have snacks in between meals, so anything outside of this set up seems out of the norm. Many people are habituated to always eating something during most times of their day. Most events we host, or attend are surrounded around food and beverages, so food is always readily available. Being without food for 16 hours sounds foreign and impossible because it is not what we are accustomed too.

Intermittent fasting brings about a new idea that life is not all about eating food all the time. People are in fear of this idea at the start, which denotes negativity; they may fail in making this big of a change due to their own negative assumptions and thoughts. Do not be afraid to be hungry, you will not starve during these 16 hours, you will survive, and be successful with weight loss, better health, and weight management.

During the beginning stages of intermittent fasting, it is vital to NOT constantly watch the clock. It is recommended that you use your time wisely. Intermittent fasting will inadvertently assist you with your time management if you listen to this recommendation. While fasting, be productive, stay busy, because 16 hours of fasting is just that 16 hours of not eating. Most people will sleep the majority of the 16 hours of fasting times, but it will take time for your body AND your mind to become accustomed to not eating breakfast or not eating or drinking whatever as soon as you wake up each morning, so make sure you attempt to stay busy and never get too much in your heard or get bored.

Some people are familiar with eating mostly junk foods. No nutrients, minerals, vitamins, or any form of a balanced meal. Sugar cravings, addictions, and food obsessiveness for these people will be one of your hardest challenges. A good way to counterbalance this is to not purchase sugary unhealthy foods to be stored near you, especially during the beginning stages of intermittent fasting. We are accustomed to snacking all the time, snacking is allowed during the feeding windows, but it is recommended to make better snack options, choose fruit, not donuts, choose whole grain cereal instead of Frosted Flakes, choose nuts over candy bars.

Your body needs to be hydrated always. Sometimes your body sends your brain signals that it's hungry when you are not physically hungry, you are instead thirsty and needing liquid intake. A major mistake is not drinking an adequate amount of water daily. To assist with making water intake routine, people can start each meal with an 8 oz glass of water, drink steeped tea during either fasting or feeding times (both are acceptable), start the morning with a glass of lemon water, and/or during the feeding windows infuse water with fruits, mints, and more.

Lastly, but in no way least of the mistakes made by beginners is the idea that you don't need to choose your foods wisely. Yes, you can eat your favorite foods, yes you can still eat out at restaurants with your families, yes you can still attend social events which includes a buffet and more, but it is recommended to choose healthier options, use portion control, and read food labels if possible; basically, make smart choices to ensure you have optimal results while intermittent fasting. There is no diet or way of eating in which you can lose weight or maintain weight with no regard to calorie intake, calories count no matter what diet or way of eating you are following. Intermittent fasting is no different, you cannot get away with excessive calorie intake.

10-Day Intermittent Fasting Routine

Described below is a sample 10-day intermittent fasting routine that can be used to help you create your own intermittent fasting daily routine schedule. This will include a fasting window to include sleeping times, feeding windows, meal options with brand name recommendations in parentheses, workout plans, and more. This sample will also include varying days in life that are not as routine to illustrate how to, even with unplanned days, intermittent fasting can still be an accomplished lifestyle for most.

Time to Decide

In my personal experience and with my research, a good starting feeding window for the 16:8 method is either 11:00 AM -7:00 PM OR from 12:00 PM -8:00 PM For the purposes of creating a 10-day sample for intermittent fasting beginners, I will use the 11:00 AM -7:00 PM feeding window for this sample. With a feeding window of 11:00 AM -7:00 PM, the fasting window is then 7:00 PM - 11:00 AM The fasting time is again the time in which you do not ingest any calories. The fasting window should go by fast since the average person will be sleeping at least 6-8 hours of the fasting window hours.

Day One

5:00 AM Gulp down 16 oz of water to awaken your system. This should be your first intake each morning.

5:30 -6:30 AM High-intensity workout like jump roping, yoga, meditation, and/or some form of physical activity. This is when you give yourself a good pep talk to endure the day. The more intense the workout the more your body will be seeking food immediately after your workout, to counterbalance this try to get as much water as possible down during your workout to trick your body into thinking you are full already.

7:00 AM Drink an 8 oz warm cup of lemon water and/or a cup of steeped tea. Tea has good antioxidants that helps the body's ability to burn more fat for fuel. Warm lemon water aids food digestion as a natural flush.

8:00 AM Drink an 8 oz cup of black coffee

9:00 AM – 11:00 AM Start work. Stay busy. Be productive. Do not get bored or be lazy. Usually, beginners will start intermittent fasting on a Sunday or Monday out of habit of trying and starting many diets previously. It's a good day, especially since its day one, the most difficult day, to meal plan and prep. Review recipes online and decide on 2-3 meals that can be planned and prepped for consumption during the rest of the week. Make a food list of items you need to pick up from the store before heading home today. This will keep you busy for a while. You will need food items for at least 3 different meal options that can be eaten as lunch or dinner, you will need some snack items and drink options.

11:00 AM First meal. This is your new norm, this is what will be known as your breakfast time:

- 2 turkey sausage patties or links (Butterball), or a few slices of bacon,
- 2 scrambled eggs, an egg while, cooked in unrefined coconut oil with spinach leaves, diced onion, tomatoes, green peppers, and turkey bacon bits,
- a protein shake (Vega) mixed with unsweetened original almond milk,
- a bottle or 2 of water

1:30 PM Fruit Time: Watermelon or Melon slices, with a glass of water

3:00 PM A serving of turkey or beef jerky and a can of sparkling water (Bubly). Some sparkling waters have artificial sweeteners, and some don't, Bubly does not. Try to choose all food and drink options that include natural ingredients mostly or all the time.

Stop by the store and pick up the items from your list. While shopping you will need maybe 2 meat options, about 4 side options (preferably fresh vegetables), waters, coffee, tea, and sparkling waters. Also, pick up other items that are healthy snacks to consume during your feeding windows between meals. Some recommended staple snack items are as follows: Fruit, veggie tray, Skinny Pop popcorn individual bags (unless you will always measure the servings before consuming), turkey/beef jerky, individual peanut butter cups, whole grain cereal, almond milk, eggs, rice cakes, nuts (individual bags), hummus, and more.

Meal prep by cooking your dinner for tonight and cooking the 2-3 meals you shopped for. Once you have cooked all the meals, use containers to package all the meals up and store in the refrigerator. If you do not have good Tupperware containers that hold a full dinner and/or lunch, it is a good idea to purchase good reusable containers and to have enough for at least 5 days. You can also use small ziplock or sandwich bags to bag up healthy snack options to always have with you when you are on the go. Go ahead and pack your lunch bag for tomorrow.

6:00 PM Final meal. 6 oz boneless skinless chicken breast seasoned and cooked in an electric skillet, with a serving of broccoli and cauliflower mix, over a small bed of brown rice, with a 16 oz bottle of water and a serving of Skinny Pop popcorn. Skinny Pop Popcorn is a favorite item because you can have 3.5 cups at a low carb, calorie, and sugar count, so it is well worth it.

7:00 PM Feeding window has closed. If you get hungry before bed drink a cup of steeped green tea with freshly squeezed lemon juice to help with fat burning during your fasting window.

Day Two & Three

5:00 AM Gulp down 16 oz of water to awaken your system

5:30 -6:30 AM High-intensity workout DVD. If you are a person who doesn't have a gym membership and doesn't want to invest in one or a trainer, you can purchase low-cost DVDs to use for exercise. Also, if you have a smart TV, you can download the YouTube app and use the many free videos available to workout in the comfort of your own home. You could also use empty space in your house or apartment to start purchasing items to have a small workout room or section in your home. Drink plenty of water.

7:00 AM Drink a warm cup of lemon water and/or a cup of steeped tea

8:00 AM Drink a cup of black coffee

9:00 AM – 11:00 AM Start work. If you get bored during this time, search the internet for Intermittent fasting transformations to pass the time, or before and after pictures, or just doing more research on intermittent fasting. Learning more and seeing results, real results will inspire you and keep you motivated, as your body works to make this a habit.

11:00 AM First meal. Eat one of your meal prepped meals, as such:

- 4 oz boneless skinless chicken breast seasoned with onions, scallions, parsley, and cilantro, topped with a hint of honey,
- Salad: Made with Spinach and Arugula as the base, 2 cut up boiled eggs, banana peppers, green peppers, onions, broccoli, carrots, bacon bits, dressed with a homemade oil and vinegar mix. Using oil and vinegar as a salad dressing saves calories for something else and adds good fats to your diet,

- a protein shake (Vega) mixed with almond milk, peanut butter, cocoa powder, half of a banana, and kale and spinach leaves
- a bottle of water or two

1:30 PM Fruit Time: A green apple with an individual cup of peanut butter, with a glass of water

3:00 PM A serving of whole grain cereal, almond milk, with cut up fresh strawberries and raspberries and a can of sparkling water (Bubly)

4:30 PM An individual bag of Emeralds cocoa dusted almonds and a handful of cashews

6:00 PM Final meal. Eat one of your meal prepped meals, as such: 6 oz wild caught lemon cream-based salmon seasoned and cooked in an electric skillet, with a serving of homemade mashed cauliflower, and a small serving of black beans, with a 16 oz bottle of water and a rice cake topped with almond butter and sliced blueberries and raspberries on top

7:00 PM Feeding window has closed. If you get hungry before bed drink a cup of steeped chamomile and lavender tea to help you rest easy tonight.

Day Four (w/ Unplanned Events)

5:00 AM Gulp down 16 oz of water to awaken your system, you could always start with more than 16 oz if your body can drink that much that early

5:30 -6:30 AM Weight training, yoga, meditation, and/or some form of physical activity. Drink plenty of water, during and after your workout to stay hydrated and avoid too much of an appetite this early.

7:00 AM Drink a warm cup of lemon water and/or a cup of steeped tea

8:00 AM Today it is your colleague's birthday and your superior calls you and ask you to stop and pick up breakfast for your department (this is an unplanned event). Choose the place with your favorite coffee and buy them breakfast (to include some fruit and whole grain options) and a jug of coffee. Your feeding window has NOT started so all you will have is a black cup of coffee and enjoy the time with your co-workers. Before everything is gone, put aside a plate of fruit and a not so sugary whole grain option for you to eat later.

9:00 AM – 11:00 AM Start work.

11:00 AM First meal. Here you can insert the breakfast you set aside for yourself this morning, which could include:

- 1 whole grain bagel with one side topped with a thin layer of cream cheese
- The plate of mixed fruit and a bag of nuts that you brought from home in your lunch bag
- And another option from your lunch box, maybe your protein shake that was prepared at home
- a bottle of water

1:30 PM a hand full of mixed nuts, string cheese, and 2 slices of rolled up turkey, with 2 glasses of water

3:00 PM A pack of raisins and a can of sparkling water (Bubly)

Unplanned event: It has now been decided that your team will leave work and head to the local bar for happy hour, with traffic you will get to the bar around 5 PM

5:00 PM If you drink it is best practice to drink liquor straight with maybe squeezes of fresh lime or lemon juice. Stop consuming additives such as agave, syrups, pre-mixed drinks, etc. Ask for a double tequila with fresh lime juice on the rocks, you can maybe have 2 of these, depending on your tolerance. Your co-workers order many appetizers to share, mostly pub food, have a bite of maybe 1 or 2 options (if you cannot totally resist) then stop and either order your food at this point OR head home to eat your already prepared food.

6:00 PM You have had 2 drinks, 2 slices of Bruschetta, 2 fried wings plain no sauce. You now decide to order and eat dinner while you are here since with traffic you won't make it home before your feeding window closes. Order like the following:

- Lettuce wrapped applewood smoked bacon burger, add a fried egg, with slices of avocado
- And a side salad instead of fries, dressed with Italian dressing
- Have a cup of black coffee before you head home

7:00 PM Feeding window has closed. If you get hungry before bed drink a cup of steeped chai tea

Day Five

5:00 AM Gulp down 16 oz of water to awaken your system

5:30 -6:30 AM if the weather is acceptable, go for a light walk/run to meditate and get physical activity at the same time. If you have a friend to join you that would be even better. This is a good time to discuss your changes so far with someone else.

7:00 AM You are exhausted and did not sleep well, drink a cup of black coffee now

8:00 AM You are still not all the way woke and/or being as productive as you would like this morning, drink another cup of black coffee

9:00 AM – 11:00 AM Start work.

11:00 AM First meal. Lunch is being served at work (Unplanned Event). Taco Day:
- Make a huge taco salad to include: lettuce, chicken and steak, black and pinto beans, sour cream, cheese, guacamole, and salsa (I say huge so you can not feel bad for excluding taco shells or tortillas)
- a bottle of fruit infused water that you prepped and brought from home
- They also brought dessert: Have a mini cupcake, you deserve it

1:30 PM Drink a cup of steeped tea with freshly squeezed lemon juice

3:00 PM A box of raisins and a handful of nuts

6:00 PM As soon as you get home, you are still so exhausted from the week you crash for a nap, which turned into you being sleep for hours (unplanned event).

9:15 PM When you wake up you realize you did not have dinner and are starving, but your feeding window has closed. Drink a cup of black decaf coffee and immediately go back to sleep.

There is a lesson in NOT having that last meal, so always be sure even if it's not a big meal you eat something before that window closes.

Day Six

5:00 AM Gulp down 16 oz of water to awaken your system

5:30 -6:30 AM You are starving because unfortunately you did not have dinner last night, so you drink a cup of black coffee early to try to fight off any unwanted appetite spikes

7:00 AM Drink the second cup of black coffee and scout the internet for intermittent fasting transformations to include real pictures of before and after results and the stories of these people

8:00 AM Force drink more water and sip a cup of hot lemon water. Try to always make sure you are using freshly squeezed lemon juice, or you can purchase the lemon juice, not from concentrate in some stores

9:00 AM – 11:00 AM Start work. Here you must stay busy, keep your mind off food, otherwise you will fail and give into temptation, as this is a long fast that you anticipated due to you not having dinner last night. Keep in mind that you will not die, some people fast for days. Some people don't eat for days because they don't have food to eat, they survive and so will you. Stay in the fight

11:00 AM First meal. Turkey burger on whole wheat pita bread, with romaine lettuce, tomatoes, mayo, mustard, and a slice of swiss cheese. A serving of BBQ kettle cooked chips, a bottle of water, and two pickle spears

1:30 PM Drink a cup of steeped tea

3:00 PM Eat 2 cups of sugar-free Jell-O

5:00 PM A bag of skinny pop and a Vega protein shake, followed by a bottle of water

6:35 PM Final meal. Have a bowl of homemade ravioli. A side salad to include spinach and romaine as the base, onions, green peppers, diced eggs, diced tomatoes, dressed with zesty Italian dressing. Dessert could be 2 scoops of dairy-free Ben and Jerrys ice-cream with a bowl of strawberries. Yes, Ben and Jerrys offers about 7 dairy-free ice cream pints, they are delicious, to say the least

7:00 PM Your feeding window has closed.

Day Seven (Weekend Plans)

9:00 AM – 10:30 AM It's the weekend, which means no work for you, so you slept in this morning. At your wake up, you awake your system with 16 oz of water. Complete one hour of weight training and a light jog on the treadmill. It is also a good time to meditate and realize you have survived 7 days of intermittent fasting.

11:00 AM First meal. 2 scrambled eggs and piece of whole grain toast. You eat light because today you are headed to a local festival that will be filled with food vendors and entertainment.

3:00 PM – 6:15 PM Cajun inspired lettuce wrapped chicken wrap, with curly fries, and water to drink. 3 straight liquor drinks mixed with lime juice, and 2 corona light bottled beers

6:15 PM 2 servings of BBQ Pulled Pork with the top slice of the bun only, with 2 small corn on the cobbs with butter, and a water to drink

7:00 PM Feeding window has closed.

9:30 PM All of your friends agree to stop and eat at a diner to finish the evening (unplanned event). You order a black decaf coffee and call it a night.

Day Eight

5:00 AM Gulp down 16 oz of water to awaken your system

5:30 -6:30 AM Meditation. Drink plenty of water.

7:00 AM Drink a warm cup of lemon water and/or a cup of steeped tea

8:00 AM Drink a cup of black coffee

9:00 AM – 11:00 AM Start work.

11:00 AM First meal.

- A Boneless, Skinless 5 oz Chicken breast, Salad Greens, Apple, and Half an Avocado
- One fruit filled cup of dairy-free yogurt, and an individual bag of nuts

1:30 PM A Can of Tuna, Apple, and 1tbs of olive oil

3:00 PM 2 individual bag of Emeralds cocoa dusted almonds

6:00 PM Final meal. Eat one of your meal prepped meals, as such:

- A serving of brown rice, spinach, and mixed vegetable medley stir fry, with ground chicken meatballs and tomato sauce, sprinkled with a little fresh parmesan cheese.

- Three or fewer cookies of your choice, depending on the food label serving size

7:00 PM Feeding window has closed. If you get hungry before bed drink a cup of steeped chamomile and lavender tea to help you rest easy tonight.

Day Nine

5:00 AM Gulp down 16 oz of water to awaken your system

5:30 -6:30 AM Hot yoga with friends. Drink plenty of water.

7:00 AM Drink a warm cup of lemon water and/or a cup of steeped tea with freshly squeezed lemon juice

8:00 AM Drink a cup of black coffee

9:00 AM – 11:00 AM Start work

11:00 AM First meal.
- 4 strips of bacon
- 3 scrambled eggs
- Whole grain toast topped with grape jelly
- Half an avocado and few slices of fresh tomatoes

1:30 PM Bowl of mixed fruit and yogurt

3:00 PM Starbucks Hot Vanilla Latte with almond milk, sugar-free vanilla, 2 Splenda, and a blueberry scone that you could not resist

6:00 PM Final meal.

- 2 Packs of Sweet and Spicy tuna on an Ole Xtreme wrap with lettuce, mayo, and tomato. Three or fewer cookies of your choice, depending on the food label serving size

7:00 PM Feeding window has closed.

Day Ten

5:00 AM Gulp down 16 oz of water to awaken your system

5:30 -6:30 AM Free group trainer session with friends. Drink plenty of water. These sessions usually burn more calories, as instead of making up your own routine, you are working with a professional who knows how to get the burn out of you

7:00 AM Drink a warm cup of lemon water and/or a cup of steeped tea to stay as hydrated as possible, because usually, trainer sessions are intense, like boot camps

8:00 AM Drink a cup of black coffee

9:00 AM – 11:00 AM Start work.

11:00 AM First meal.
- 4 strips of bacon
- An omelet to include: 2 eggs, 2 egg whites, spinach, kale, onions, red and green peppers, broccoli, and fresh tomatoes
- Half of a whole grain croissant with grape jelly
- Half an avocado

1:30 PM Bowl of mixed fruit, yogurt, and a handful of cashew nuts

3:00 PM Starbucks Iced Vanilla Latte with almond milk, sugar-free vanilla, 2 Splenda, heavy cream, and 2 chocolate chip cookies

6:00 PM Final meal.

- Pulled chicken tortilla soup
- 2 fried avocado taco's
- Chicken tinga burrito
- A serving of grilled shrimp on the side

7:00 PM Feeding window has closed.

Changing it Up

How to Turn Any Diet into the 16:8 Method

The 16:8 Intermittent Fasting Method can work well with any other diet or way of eating you are already on. Most other diets are geared around restricting certain food groups or food with certain ingredients, but not intermittent fasting. Intermittent fasting does not restrict any food group, it is created this way, so you can eat your favorite foods, as long as they are eaten within the designated feeding window, and as long as you are fasting, during the designated fasting window

For those who are vegan, vegetarian, paleo, pescatarian, etc., you can still exclude what you want and still intermittent fast. To do this, eat the same way you are eating now, but these foods must be eaten within your feeding window, and you must fast within your fasting window. Nothing else must change, only the timing of your eating. For those who are low carbers, keto, weight watchers, gluten free, grain free, etc., you can still exclude what you want and include only what is allowed and still intermittent fast. To do this, you eat the same foods, drink the same drinks, and exclude what is required, you just only eat during your feeding window, and fast only during your fasting window.

An intermittent fasting vegan could have a feeding window of 10 AM-6 PM. With this you can have a vegan meal at 10 AM, Vegan snacks at 1 PM, Vegan Shake at 3 PM, and your last Vegan Meal at 5:35 PM. This illustrates that you can still be vegan and intermittent fast. This is only an example for vegans, but others can use this same plan, others like paleo eaters, vegetarians, dairy free people, gluten free people, and more.

An intermittent fasting person who is also gluten and dairy free as a consequence of health issues, also works over night as a nurse, this person feeding window may be from 11 PM to 7 AM. With this feeding window and way of eating he/she may have 3 portioned meals at 11 PM, 2 AM, and 6:30 AM, all while ensuring their meals are dairy and gluten free. As you can see, their way of eating and not eating did not have to change, only the timing of eating these meals.

An intermittent fasting keto person could increase their fats, proteins, and dairy as keto people do, as long as they are only eating during that feeding window. This persons feeding window could be from 9 AM to 5 PM. This person could have a LCHF (low carb high fat) meal at 9 AM and 4PM and the appropriate keto snacks in between.

Time management is the principal to be successful with intermittent fasting. You can exclude food groups that you want, you can include food groups that you want, you can restrict your carbs, you can restrict your calories, you can exercise or not exercise, and still be successful with intermittent fasting. The uniqueness of intermittent fasting makes it even more amazing than any other way of eating. The USDA recommends NOT restricting important food groups, so everyone should be willing to at least try it once or twice, if needed.

The Intermittent Fasting Lifestyle

Monitor & Assess Progress

If you are starting intermittent fasting to not only improve your health, but to also lose weight it is very important to take your initial weight, take measurements, and take pictures before you begin.

Scale Weigh-Ins

The morning of day 1 it is important to get on the scale either nude or in very little clothes. It is important to weigh yourself before eating or drinking anything. Choose a time and weigh yourself, this will be known as your starting weight. It is important that you not only weigh yourself but to also write this number down and/or enter it into your phone or an app that you are using to keep track of your progress. I think it's better for you to write it down in a journal along the way so you can see your progress in real time side by side.

It may also be a good idea to calculate your Body Mass Index (BMI) and your Body Fat Percentage, there are apps to calculate both, or a simple google search can result in free calculators to get this information. To prevent my scale victories from being non-victories, I choose the same day and time to weigh myself, once a week, only once a week. While intermittent fasting, you will lose inches faster than you will lose pounds from the scale, it is very important that you understand that, so that you don't get discouraged and quit. Therefore, I recommend to not only weigh yourself but to also take measurements and pictures to always see what progress you have made.

Measurement Tracking

The morning of day 1 it is important to take your measurements. You will need to buy a measuring tape to have on hand. I purchased one in my favorite color to make me feel better about myself while taking the measurements. It is important to measure yourself before eating or drinking anything. Choose a time and measure yourself, this will be known as your starting measurements. It is important that you not only measure yourself but to also write these numbers down and/or enter it into your phone or an app that you are using to keep track of your progress. I think it's better for you to write it down in a journal along the way so you can see your progress in real time side by side.

I usually take the following measurements: neck circumference, waist, hips, arms, thigh, bust, belly pouch, and calf. You can measure more or less. I take 3 separate measurements from my waist and stomach area, because feel like its 3 separate body parts. I take measurements at the same time each day and week that I weigh myself.

Before & After

The morning of day 1 it is important to take before pictures, so you have proof of how you looked on day 1. It is important to take your pictures before eating or drinking anything. Choose a time and get used to taking these pictures yourself, as someone may not always be around to help you with this (the same thing for your measurements, do this yourself), this will be known as your before picture.

I usually take pictures from all angles: front, back, both sides, one with a flexed muscle, etc., whichever pictures you decide to take do those same pictures each time you take pictures. This along with how my clothes fit is the tell all of what is really progressing and what is not or still needs work. Once, I have my pictures taken, I then use different apps to create collages to see the progress of the latest picture with the newest picture. I spend hours reviewing every inch of my body on these pictures to make sure I see all my victories. This is the best way to track your weight loss progress.

Hacks to Success

There are many principal tips and tricks that I use till this day to continue to ensure my success. While intermittent fasting is all about the timing of your meals and fasting, it can be so much more if you decide to use all the resources available to you to keep it exciting, continue to learn new things, be creative, be consistent and prepare and be prepared always. Intermittent fasting along with the hacks discussed below will change your weight and your life forever.

Sharing is Caring

I am not certain if this will help anyone other than myself or not, but it did help and is still helping me. I have learned that I am best at all things in life when I am helping others along the way. I have been sharing my knowledge with people day in and day and have become a coach of intermittent fasting to many. By encouraging others, I have simultaneously helped myself, because it's a shame to teach what you can't follow right? I won't be that type of coach. I practice what I am teaching. Me writing this book has helped me learn that I know so much about this topic, which is why I have been so much more successful this time around.

I gain so much pleasure from my social media followers interest in my story and growth. I have so much respect from my coworkers and friends and they all ask so much questions about IF, so literally this is all I talk about, which is fine by me, it holds me accountable. I don't want to let myself down to include a lot of people who are seamlessly watching me out of the corner of their eyes. I am helping someone else with this knowledge, which helps me.

Apps to Download

Pinterest is such a good resource to use when it comes to planning meals to keep eating the healthier way. This app includes links to recipes, grocery lists, meal idea, how to prep these meals, and more. YouTube, of course, is a great resource to review other people's struggles, peaks, and pits, before and after pictures, to hear their stories, to help you stay motivated and understand that most of what you go through while attempting to make this a habit, others have gone through the same things. MyFitnessPal's blog and community sections of its app is another great resource to use to join communities that are specific to intermittent fasting and all its components

These are good apps to have downloaded on your mobile device, iPad, or tablet. Using all your free time on these apps should be your new hobby instead of scrolling on your social media, especially since everything you see and hear will contribute to the success of making intermittent fasting a hobby.

Food Delivery Services

Some people decide that Meal Planning and Meal Prep is just not a realistic lifestyle for them. They may live a busier life than average, have a big active family, hate to cook, can't cook, don't want to cook, hate shopping, not creative, and more reasons. These people may choose to use a meal planning/prep or food delivery service to assist them with their meals.

Sometimes this can be costly, sometimes it may be affordable, but what it is, is convenient and by using this service you are still preparing in advance for what life throws at you during this change. You are still choosing healthier options, and being creative in what you eat.

Journaling

This lifestyle change will change your life forever. One day you will have changed so much that you may want to share your journey with others. If you decide to share, what better way to share than to go back and see how you felt each day or a few days. It is best practice to journal while you go through this journey. Journaling can be helpful in discovering what your negative triggers are, tracking your weight and measurement progress, tracking your feelings towards food, tracking your growth toward meal planning and food shopping and eating out and chosen food options, tracking your every step along the way. Your first journal entry should note why you are doing IF and explain your goals.

Sometimes people go as far as to go back to school for nutrition, or to be a trainer, life coach, and more, this journal will only assist you in tracking it all in real time. Your journal could be the road to success for someone or some other people who feel as though you once felt. This can also help you when you have those hard days and want to give up, you can read back and know that I was feeling like this once before and overcame it so surely, I can again. Journaling can only help you on this journey, it is best practice for success.

Family Lifestyle Change

I wouldn't recommend making a drastic change, but after a few days maybe a week it's a good idea to start your family and sometimes even the company you keep around you to start eating what you eat and when you eat. If you are the cook and shopper in your house, this will be a better use of your time. You will only have to meal plan once, shop once, and cook a few meals that will feed everyone for a couple of days. Hopefully, this gives you more time during the week to add in exercise if you don't, or if you do maybe a second workout, or maybe give you a few hours of time each day to do something else you have been wanting to do, like maybe writing a book.

Brush your Teeth Earlier

Everyone should brush their teeth before bed each night. With intermittent fasting, it's better to practice brushing your teeth after your last meal. The taste of toothpaste and/or Listerine should keep you from wanting to do any further eating. This is just a mind trick, but it has been a successful helpful trick that I still use.

How to Order at Restaurants

Know the menu before you go. I repeat, know the menu before you go. Most restaurants, even fast food restaurants, have websites in which you can view their menu options. If you know what's on the menu before you go, you can be proactive in deciding what you will order as the best option for you. Have a few staple times that most restaurants offer: grilled salmon, chicken breast, shrimp, any seafood, fried chicken wings no breading or sauce, burgers wrapped in lettuce, salads, and more.

Most restaurants DO NOT serve appropriate portions of food. This is an advertising mechanism for the restaurants, it is an effective way for them to get you to continually come back and spend money with them. I mean who wants to go to a restaurant that serves those small plate options. Most restaurants serve 2 and sometimes 3 times the portion that a person should be eating in one sitting.

To ensure you spend your money wisely but getting the food you pay for, while simultaneously ensuring that you are using good portion control, when you order at a restaurant it is good practice to go ahead and ask for a to-go plate and when your food arrives, split your food up by keeping an appropriate portion to eat now and package away the other 2 or 3 servings for later options.

Lunch Bag Prep

Every evening after dinner, clean the kitchen and prepare for the next day. This includes preparing my lunch bag for the next day. I add the following to my lunch bag each day. 2 full meals, 3-4 snacks, and 2-3 bottles of water and a sparkling water. Although most days, I eat dinner at home, what if I didn't make it home in time to eat dinner, or what if football practice goes long, what if traffic is a mess due to an accident, what if I must work late, what if, what if, what if. Always be prepared and you will be successful. I have had unplanned events, which have forced me to eat in the car, and sometimes dinner is a few healthy snacks because I didn't have my meal with me. Be prepared.

How to Deal with Unplanned Events

Although unplanned life events occur, sometimes 3-4 times a week, as an intermittent faster you still need to have a plan for the unplanned. Always have that lunch box/bag with you as previously mentioned. Know a few staple food options that are your go-to food options when you are on the go and don't have your own available food options. Think before you eat always.

Peer pressure is real, especially at social events, be sure to have a serious conversation with family and friends so they know you are serious and that they should not offer you items when it is not your feeding window and that your new lifestyle is not a joking matter and that you would appreciate they take it as an important part of your life. Make good decisions and be proud of those decisions that you make. Every now and then, I change my feeding windows for social events. I sometimes fast longer so that I can push my feeding window back to be able to attend social events and have dinner and drinks with family and friends.

Buy in Bulk

You may be thinking how is buying in buck related to intermittent fasting. It is vital for beginner and sometimes long time intermittent fasters to always have food on hand to accommodate any cravings and their feeding windows. It is best practice to buy favorite snack foods in bulk if available. When you buy these items in bulk you can then use small ziplock and/or sandwich bags to create your own individual serving size (according to the food label) baggies to keep in your car, purse, backpack, at school, at work, in your gym bag, in your lunch box or bag, and more.

It saves you money to buy in bulk than to buy individual items already prepackage, companies charge more for convenience, so when you buy prepackaged small cute individually packaged items it costs more than buying in bulk and doing this yourself. This also ensures that you are only having a serving or 2 according to the food label. This also saves you from not being prepared and eating unplanned food items.

Consistent Routine

Appetite is trainable because it is driven by routine. Our bodies know and learn our routines, we are usually hungry when we expect to be hungry, not necessarily when we are physically hunger, again it could be that we are bored or need fluids. Practice makes perfect, right? Fasting is a skill that with intermittent fasting you are trying to advance this skill.

Best practice would be at least start with a good routined new life as you endure this lifestyle change. That means set your alarm and wake to start most days at the same time, specifically during the week to start. Eat your first meal and 2nd meal at the same times, you can have your snacks at whatever time during the feeding window. It is also best practice to workout at the same time of the day most days and take measurements, pictures, and weigh yourself on these same days. Meal plan the week before you will shop and cook the meals. Then shop on the same day, and cook and prep the meals on the same day so you start the week always with good habits.

Setbacks

Setbacks are sometimes inevitable when it comes to any type of life change, intermittent fasting is no different. Setbacks can include general fasting knowledge, lack of discipline, willpower, self-control, fear of missing out, lack of planning or procrastination, illnesses, that may or may not include medications, that prevent this type of fasting, lack of motivation, resistance to change, YOU, and much more.

YOU

You will be your biggest setback, challenge, and critic during this attempt to change. Many people have issues with confidence, self-esteem, feeling deserving, discipline, consistency, peer pressure, unawareness, and more, which ALL can contribute to YOU being your worst nightmare during this change and ultimately maybe your demise in many aspects of life.

You must realize you are the only person who can make a change in your life, and that goes for all changes you want to make. You are responsible for your own happiness and if changing your eating lifestyle is what will make you happier, then this information gives you the knowledge to be able to make this change without help from anyone else. YOU can make this change happen for YOU, and only you. You should be beginning this journal to please only you and not just for appearance purposes, but for through and through happiness and well-being.

You must believe in yourself. You must know that you are your #1 priority and must be your biggest supporter. If no one else cares, you must care enough to change your habits and be consistent in the changes you decide to make. No one should be able to derail you from making such an important change in your life.

You are responsible for your choices. This is a LIFEstyle change so if you mess up, just do better the next time, don't quit on yourself. Don't make decisions based on temporary needs or feelings, think about what you do as you do it to make decisions that are better for you overall in the future. Think about your future, do you want to be trying another diet in another 30 days? Do you still want to be in the same body with the same health in 30 days? Would you rather feel comfortable in your clothes and skin and feel healthy throughout?

Practice Makes Perfect

Getting acquainted with the process of fasting in general and testing your chosen time frames for your feeding and fasting windows can be a difficult time if you are used to eating many meals/snacks daily. Being motivated to continue to develop in this change is just as important as anything else that comes along with this change. Live each day separately, as in if something did not go to your liking one day, change your process the next until you have feeding and fasting windows that work well with your daily routine schedule. Mind over matter, you matter, so make sure your mind continues to know this fact to ensure you aren't resistant to this change.

Don't be Weak

During the initial change stage, there must be an increased amount of willpower, discipline, and self-control. You will be required to practice your self-control around others who are NOT on an intermittent fasting lifestyle. A person needs to have the willpower to refrain from ingesting calories during their fasting window. You need to have the discipline to create these time frames and stick to them, and when the feeding and/or fasting windows are broken, create consequences for yourself to ensure it does not happen again until it does not happen anymore.

Fear of Missing Out (FOMO)

Because of how you are used to living your life, sometimes you may feel like you are missing out on the fun surrounding social and/or family eating events, but consider the fact that you are making this change to perfect how you feel and how you look to ensure you are around for a long life to enjoy life. Family and friends may not be on this lifestyle and either will or will not support this change. Alcohol should be consumed in moderation. If you choose to drink alcohol, two or less daily drinks should be the max. Choose non-sugary spirits and alcohol volume dry wines to ensure you are getting the best buzz for your choice.

Holidays will more than likely be the biggest change for you and the biggest day to test you when new to this lifestyle. Holidays are all about eating and tasting everything with family and friends and making memories. Try to prepare in advance by either assisting with cooking to ensure meals are ready before/during your feeding window and choose your favorites to ensure you are satisfied and not as vulnerable after your feeding window closes. The holidays will test you.

Prepare, Don't Procrastinate

Preparation is key. Now that you have decided on your feeding window, ALWAYS, make sure you have your meals/snacks readily available during these times. Stay ahead of your schedule a day or so, to ensure you pack your meals/snacks if you will be away from home when it is time to eat those meals/snacks to ensure. Even if you plan to be home, always make sure you take at least a few snack options with your wherever you go, by preparing in this way you ensure not to ever get caught out and about for hours with nothing to eat just wasting your feeding window away.

Not Reading Labels and Controlling Portions

Although your calories are NOT restricted when intermittent fasting, eating too much of even healthy foods can lead to weight gain no matter the type of diet/lifestyle you are following. To prevent this type of setback meal plan, use portion control, be consistent with choosing the most nutritious food choices, and measure your foods to ensure you are not eating too many servings in one meal.

Nonsense from Others

There are times in life when it's better to keep your goals to yourself. Keep your goals away from negative people, specifically keep negative people away from your goals and out of your life. To be successful in many things in life, you need a support system, which does not include negative people. You need someone who can cheer you on, someone who can motivate you, someone, who may be willing to join you, someone who doesn't add to your problems by persuading you to do what is against your goals. If you have these types of people in your life, do not tell them your plan of intermittent fasting.

Many people have their own preconceived assumptions about fasting, and intermittent fasting, and usually their views are without researched knowledge and education. It is important that you understand and know myth versus facts when it comes to intermittent fasting. People who have tried all types of diets, seem to think they know them all, and they are very discouraging at times. During a lifestyle change as intermittent fasting, it is very easy to get discouraged, so stay the course and keep those people away, while you try this out yourself based on your researched facts.

Myths vs. Facts

Understanding the differences is important to your success. Myths may create too much negative space and create room for failure. Facts should educate you enough to keep you motivated and interested in proving that you can be successful with intermittent fasting. It is a myth that not eating 5-6 meals a day will ruin your metabolism and muscle mass. It is a myth that intermittent fasting causes muscle loss, encourages overeating, causes food cravings, causes nutrient deficiencies, and is unnatural and unhealthy for your body. It is a fact that intermittent fasting creates consistencies in eating habits, helps with fat loss and weight management, and promotes a healthy system. Myths are generally kept alive for financial interest.

The Dreaded Scale

Weighing yourself daily is normal for some people, especially those who have tried so many diets, fads, supplements, diet drinks, food restrictions, etc. so this won't be any different. It is normal to want to weigh yourself daily, but this is not healthy for the success of living an intermittent fasting lifestyle. Weigh yourself one day out of the week, same day, same time, same platform and place of scale, same clothes or no clothes, etc. Weighing yourself should be part of your routine. Choose a day and time and stick to it, BUT don't get too caught up on numbers.

Intermittent fasting burns fat as fuel so the scale may not move as fast as you would expect, but to counterbalance this, you will be losing continues measurements, so be sure to take your measurements and pictures of yourself from all angles. Don't let the numbers on the scale be the thing that makes you quit intermittent fasting, observe the fitting of your clothes, keep note of your measurements and look at how your numbers drop, and create grids of before and after pictures to compare your weight success.

Social Media

It's very easy to get caught up on what you see and read on social media. The many transformation stories are fabulous and sound to simple, easy, and those before and after pictures, are like heaven to your eyes. You see that one person that you are following who's before picture looks just like you currently, and you wonder. Why haven't I gotten there? Why did it only take her 3 months to look like this? What am I doing wrong? Am I doing anything right? Is my process working? Is intermittent fasting having any positive effects for me?

A million questions will enter your mind. Some people do tell their stories, but most people tell the best of their stories and not the struggle that people have usually been having for years. Don't let anything from anyone else on social media or in passing be the reason you have setbacks or quit on this new journey. You can do this.

Illnesses

Lastly, illness could be considered a potential temporary setback, or even sometimes permanent. If this occurs, please see your medical professional on advice on how to move forward with this change or not, depending on what is recommended, sometimes it may just be a change in times or a similar change.

The Lifestyle Change and Daily Routine

Creating Habits

There is a huge adaptive component needed to be successful in changing your lifestyle to include intermittent fasting. The most important aspect is learning to create a habit, being consistent regardless of what life has to offer for you. Habits are hard to create. To create a habit, write down your daily routine and stick with it. Share your daily routine with family members to ensure they know what your new routine consists of and what it does not include. Commit to at least 21 days initial to make the habits and routine stick and make it as simple as possible.

Your response to things is what creates habits. With intermittent fasting, it is critical that during your fasting windows, if you get hungry or have cravings, that you gravitate to water, coffee, and tea, this response will become an effective response to hunger, which will create a successful habit to maintain intermittent fasting.

Skipping Days

As you begin to attempt to create habits, skipping days of intermittent fasting is not effective. Once you start this change, it is critical that regardless of weekends, holidays, social events, and more that you make this routine so that your habits begin to stick. Skipping days restarts the process for your body and mind and restarting intermittent fasting continuous is NOT a habit that you are sticking too. You must be consistent. There is no positive to put your mind and/or body through this repeatedly without committing to making it a habit.

Old Habits Die Hard

Yes, they do. Eating habits are developed in your childhood. You may not realize it, but you may still be eating like a child, as your parents taught you. I was still eating all my food from my plate when I initially started intermittent fasting. By completely devouring all my food, I realized I was not eating proportionately and was always overeating, which was one of the main issues within my old eating habits. You can eat all the healthy foods you want, but if you are overeating those foods and not using portion control, you will not lose weight, nor will you maintain weight, you will continually gain weight. This was a very big win for me when I finally discovered this and acted.

Try to observe how you eat, what you eat, when you eat, what you are doing when you eat, some aspects regarding your food relationship may be done subconsciously, and only by being very observant you can take note of certain actions and start making effective changes to be successful with intermittent fasting. Kill these old habits by any means necessary, to do that observe yourself always and figure out why you are the way you are, how are you, how can you change you and your relationship with food for the better. Change your variables to make intermittent fasting work for you.

Make it Simple

To make this a simple change, decide on your feeding and fasting windows as close to your life schedule now. Create a few meals and snack options and stick to a limited list, to begin with for meal planning and shopping; don't have too many options. Too many options could make this change seem impossible when it doesn't have to be, so keep everything simple. You don't have to journal every day if you don't just automatically gravitate to it. You don't have to measure foods and meal preps all the time, do what you can when you can, don't put too much pressure on anything.

Conclusion

With our intermittent fasting approach and now the success, we, as a couple, were able to conceive naturally and have our first child. With that fact alone, intermittent fasting has changed my life forever and made me the happiest self that I could ever be. I am extremely happy I came across what is known as Intermittent Fasting. With the so much access to the world wide web, there was tons of information to educate me on this lifestyle approach; this information guided me in so many ways and assisted me with changing my eating habits to fit my lifestyle, while also making it the best life ever.

With my success with intermittent fasting, I am no longer pre-diabetic and am in the best health of my lifetime. My body fat percentage is lower, my weight is lower, my BMI (body mass index) is much lower, I can see my abs, I have toned arms and legs, my feet size even went down (she says her bra size went down as well, which too some could be a positive or negative). I feel better. I look better. I sleep better. My clothes fit me better. And I and my family are better together.

The changes I was able to make to my own life while intermittent fasting have been super rewarding. It was also a very hard change to make, it was very difficult at first, but it taught me a lot about myself, and if I put my mind to something, no matter what it is, I can make anything happen. If I can make this change, and succeed with intermittent fasting, anyone can. That anyone includes YOU. You have to choose yourself first, you have to make yourself a priority, you have to never give up on yourself, you have to know that you are worthy, you have to know that you deserve this change, you have to WANT happiness and you have to go get that happiness for yourself. No one is more responsible for your happiness and success than you are.

Happiness comes with feeling good inside and out. Happiness comes with looking good to others, as well as, yourself. Happiness comes when you realize you have made hard decisions to better your life by being consistent and sticking to those decisions. Happiness comes when you are at optimal health and everyone, includes yourself, sees a change in you for the better. Happiness is yours, if you want it. Intermittent fasting can be step one to you becoming as happy as you want to be.

To show gratitude to intermittent fasting, I continue to spread the word about this great lifestyle. I am now an author, public speaker, and now training to be a nutritionist. Presently, I am still intermittent fasting each day. I am using the same feeding and fasting times, and I eat healthier and healthier each day as I educate myself more and more. I am a lean mean fat fighting machine, that eats my favorite foods whenever I want.

References

[14] American Diabetes Association. (2015, August 13). The Best Food Choices. Retrieved from http://www.diabetes.org/food-and-fitness/weight-loss/food-choices/the-best-food-choices/

[13] American Heart Association. (2018, April 18). American Heart Association Recommendations for Physical Activity for Adults. Retrieved from http://www.heart.org/en/healthy-living/fitness/fitness-basics/aha-recs-for-physical-activity-in-adults

[10] Berkhan, Martin. (2010, April 14). The Leangains Guide. Retrieved from https://leangains.com/the-leangains-guide/

[11] Collier, R. (2013). Intermittent fasting: the science of going without. CMAJ : Canadian Medical Association Journal, 185(9), E363–E364. http://doi.org/10.1503/cmaj.109-4451

[7, 9] Department of Health and Human Services and U.S. Department of Agriculture. 2015-2020 Dietary Guidelines for Americans. 8th ed. December 2015. Retrieved from health.gov/dietaryguidelines/2015/resources/2015-2020_Dietary_Guidelines.pdf.

[8] Food Allergy Research and Education. (n.d.). Milk Allergy. Retrieved October 15, 2018, from https://www.foodallergy.org/common-allergens/milk

[15] Hallböök, T., Ji, S., Maudsley, S., & Martin, B. (2012). The effects of the ketogenic diet on behavior and cognition. Epilepsy Research, 100(3), 304–309. http://doi.org/10.1016/j.eplepsyres.2011.04.017

[3] Harvard T.H. Chan School of Public Health. (n.d.). *Diet Review: Intermittent Fasting for Weight Loss.* Retrieved from https://www.hsph.harvard.edu/nutritionsource/healthy-weight/diet-reviews/intermittent-fasting/

[4] Krikorian, R., Shidler, M. D., Dangelo, K., Couch, S. C., Benoit, S. C., & Clegg, D. J. (2012). Dietary ketosis enhances memory in mild cognitive impairment. Neurobiology of Aging, 33(2), 425.e19–425.e27. http://doi.org/10.1016/j.neurobiolaging.2010.10.006

[5] Longo, V. D., & Panda, S. (2016). Fasting, circadian rhythms, and time restricted feeding in healthy lifespan. Cell Metabolism, 23(6), 1048–1059. http://doi.org/10.1016/j.cmet.2016.06.001

[17] Martin, Laura J. (2016, August 22). How to read food labels. Retrieved from https://medlineplus.gov/ency/patientinstructions/000107.htm

[12] National Institute of Diabetes and Digestive and Kidney Diseases. (n.d.). Diet and Nutrition. Retrieved October 13, 2018, from https://www.niddk.nih.gov/health-information/diet-nutrition

[1, 2, 6] Patterson, R. E., Laughlin, G. A., Sears, D. D., LaCroix, A. Z., Marinac, C., Gallo, L. C., ... Villaseñor, A. (2015). INTERMITTENT FASTING AND HUMAN METABOLIC HEALTH. Journal of the Academy of Nutrition and Dietetics, 115(8), 1203–1212. http://doi.org/10.1016/j.jand.2015.02.018

[16] Tello, Monique. (2018, June 29). *Intermittent fasting: Surprising update.* Retrieved from https://www.health.harvard.edu/blog/intermittent-fasting-surprising-update-2018062914156

The Keto Lifestyle

Simple 7 Day Meal Plans To Kickstart Your Ketogenic Diet

By

Mary Parrett

Introduction

More often than not, engaging and persevering in laborious performances to keep you fit and trim would seem to become exasperating. In the end, you will only come to realize that everything you do never makes any sense. Rather than achieving your weight-loss goals, you eventually lose all your patience!

Besides, the several varieties of weight-loss programs dominating in the fitness world today, yet, passing as fleeting fads, only confuse you even more. Additionally, when you cope up strictly with their program guidelines, they only entail great difficulties.

As a resolve, the **THE KETO LIFESTYLE** presents incisively the ketogenic or keto diet as your ultimate solution. Foremost, the meal plans demonstrated herein will be your invaluable strategies on how to control your caloric intakes, promote enhanced fat-burning and metabolic processes in your body, boost the growths of lean muscle mass, or shed off your excessive and unwanted kilos while staying fit in the quickest, safest, and healthiest way possible.

Lest you think warily that this book has a catch, the meal plans and the diet itself will even tolerate you to consume more fats! Yes, you have just read it right—you eat FAT to keep you FIT!

While this may sound like science fiction, you must better believe it. The fat-ness for fitness eating plan is not a myth, and it will never be! It is actually part of the natural metabolic calisthenics of the body. In other words, it is the healthiest alternative that your body necessitates. See for yourself after digesting further the meat of the matter!

Essentially, the unorthodox ketogenic regimen is exclusively a low-carbohydrate and high-fat diet. Vegetable and animal oils, butter, and heavy cream are the usual components in your keto meal plans to provide you with the necessary fats. Therefore, such fats will be the reason for letting you shy away from taking sweets (sugar or glucose-based carbohydrates).

By simply replacing basic carbohydrates with healthy fats, the regimen eventually transforms your body into a virtual fat-burning machine! Hence, since your body will be burning fewer carbohydrates, your cognitive processes heighten because your brain uses up more stored fats for energy; and in no time than you will expect, your appetite decreases, which results in dramatic losses in body weight!

While the keto dietary program restricts strictly carbohydrate-rich foods, it can still allow you to accept generous levels of tolerances. Nonetheless, you ought to measure your meals accordingly in terms of the diet's ideal daily macronutrient intakes or calorie consumptions.

Apparently, you may be forming doubts and misgivings about the regimen by all its specific food restrictions and tolerances. Yet, on the contrary, the old perception that fats are harmful to your health is now fast becoming a yarn. This no longer imposes any precautions with the diet.

Therefore, you can really rule out any thoughts of food deprivation. Besides, you can still feast on your favorite foods while enrolled in the program since you will have several alternatives for their essential ingredients that are as delectable, yet, healthier.

Medical research and science have been helping us to improve our basic understandings of proper nutrition. At this point, we must have already learned that many types of fats can truly be healthy for the body! For all we know, fats definitely manifest major improvements in various health risk factors such as cholesterol and blood sugar levels. Fact is that the keto dietary plan continuously provides a myriad of time-tested health and wellness benefits.

For this reason, several new variations and tweaked adaptations of the keto diet mushroomed but merely flourished as short-lived trends. Generally, they capitalized more on the marketing ploy of weight reduction but compromised the significance of staying fit and healthy.

The Atkins diet, which is also a low-carbohydrate and high fat (LCHF) diet, has been one of the most notable versions of these modifications. However, the only distinctive difference is that the ketogenic diet regulates moderate protein consumptions. In short, it actually focuses to control each macronutrient intake. At any rate, you can then consider the ketogenic diet as an instituted dietary discipline that is more holistic with its working principles and basic concept.

Hereupon these pages contain your fundamental guide towards a deeper understanding of the keto diet. They primarily direct you to learn the principle of attaining the natural and ideal metabolic state of the body through optimal ketosis. Moreover, the book aims to distinguish the keto regimen as an established medical nutrition therapy for eating more fats in order to lose weight. All the information you gained from this book will prepare you towards the proper performances and implementations of the diet.

First, you will know how to calculate for your recommended calorie intake values. These values will be significant in shaping to create your food recipes and meal plans, and eventually, help you stay on course with the diet.

Second, you will have a definite grocery guide of recommended and restricted food groups to help you stick to the regimen. This also enables you to form prudent decisions on choosing your ideal keto meal.

Third, the book provides you with 80 inspiring, delicious, budget-friendly, and easy-to-prepare keto recipes categorized under breakfast, lunch, dinner, snack, and dessert meals. Each recipe will comprise the 7-day meal plan samples across 1,500-, 1,750-, and 2,000- calorie consumptions. Hence, the book covers the range of your healthy weight goals and wellness agenda depending on your recommended or calculated daily calorie consumption.

Exciting as it could ever be, you will most likely have your moments of glory for whipping up your personal recipes or formulating other food preparation variations as soon as you get the hang of practicing the ketogenic diet! You only have to trust and live by the process!

Chapter 1-Knowing Deeper the Ketogenic Diet

Originally, the popular indulgence of the keto diet was for patients afflicted with epilepsy and seizures. However, no one could really determine precisely the working mechanisms of the diet in alleviating or treating seizures. Despite all the formulated theories on how the diet works, the definite assurance for its neurological therapeutic values is the occurrence of metabolic changes that greatly influence the brain's chemical composition.

During the recent past, the keto diet has regained new interests due to its slew of therapeutic potentials. The medical field affirms its feasibility for treating patients diagnosed with diabetes and cancer, as well as people suffering from neurodegenerative diseases, like Alzheimer's disease, Parkinson's disease, and brain damage during a stroke.

In 1921, Dr. Russell Wilder of the Mayo Clinic in Minnesota developed the ketogenic diet, which focuses on a very low consumption of carbohydrates and a high intake of fats. The ketogenic diet derived its terminology from *ketogenesis*, which is the metabolic process of generating sufficient quantities of ketone bodies. This process is a natural alternative function of our body's metabolism that allows us to survive without food intakes for a definite period.

With this specific eating habit, the diet produces a similar effect on fasting, whereby, the body ultimately creates ketone bodies in the liver. During fasting, the level of glucose in the blood decreases (hypoglycemia). Glucose is the major nutrient of muscles, especially the brain. The body would then adapt itself to the deprivation of food, as well as the reduction of glucose by tapping its reserves of energy. Typically, the body draws in the stored fatty tissues, which the liver transforms into ketone bodies.

On average, your body can store hundreds of thousands of calories, which comprise of fats. Thus, your liver produces large quantities of ketone bodies during fasting. After three days into the fast, the energy at the level of neuron cells in the nervous system will be a third of ketone bodies. This denotes that your body will seemingly have an unlimited supply of energy. It now only depends on how long you sustain living through without food. Unfortunately, therefore, a complete fasting plan leads to muscle loss; and obviously, it could not be a feasible and lasting healthy solution.

Under the ketogenic diet, the ketone bodies—sourced from the metabolism or breaking down of fat intakes—enable all your body cells (including neurons) to be functionally flexible. With higher fat and lower carbohydrate consumption, your body incurs lower glucose levels over time. The erstwhile glucose-reliant cells of your body switch automatically to burning ketone bodies for fuel.

Ketone bodies possess uniquely desirable characteristics. In comparison to glucose, burning ketones result in lesser oxidative damages to your cells. In fact, the brain and heart function better with energy sourced from ketone bodies rather than glucose. As such, this also implies that ketones are more effective in generating greater energy than the body does from burning glucose. Hence, ketones are much efficient, safer, and healthier body fuels for your cells to use.

Program Principles & Core Concept

Ketogenesis normally occurs to all of us, particularly when we fast, skip a meal, or simply, lower our carbohydrate or glucose intakes. The minimum lifetime carbohydrate limit seems to be zero, especially if we consume adequate amounts of proteins and fats.[1] It is, therefore, a completely natural state that has allowed humanity to thrive through millennia.

This indicates that ketogenesis suppresses our appetite without experiencing the gnawing pangs of hunger or fasting. Therefore, engaging with a diet rich in fats, yet, less in carbohydrates promotes ketogenesis.

Your principal purpose now in indulging with the ketogenic diet is how to govern your body cells into mobilizing its natural alternative function of shifting into the metabolic process of ketogenesis. This simply means that you should attain a state of optimal ketosis—**switching your body's main metabolic function from the processing of carbohydrates to the breaking down of fats to produce ketone bodies for fuel.**

In terms of reducing weight, the reduction of carbohydrate intakes is a given and well established. The ketogenic diet is no exception. Not only will the diet allow you to lose weight easily but also, it helps to alter or reverse effectively health risk factors often linked to chronic heart disease (CHD) and diabetes such as *glycemia* (concentrated presence of glucose along the bloodstream), blood *triglycerides* (bad cholesterol in the blood), and various symptoms of inflammatory diseases [2, 0, 0, 0, 0].

Attaining Optimal Ketosis = A-OK!

Switching your body quickly into an optimal state of ketosis heavily depends on your food consumption! High-fat diets are effective for the simple reason that they force your body to trigger undergoing a state of ketosis.

Ketosis is actually a metabolic state wherein your body has an extremely high fat-burning rate. During this state, ketone bodies in your blood begin to increase exponentially. Obviously, your body has no carbohydrates to burn primarily except fats!

Oftentimes, many adherents to the strict ketogenic regimen become very cautious and conscious that their ketone levels in the blood might fall beyond the ideal values. This should not surprise you. **The key to the proper performance of the diet is to avoid all foods derived from starchy sources, or plainly, carbohydrates! You should be restrictive on your carbohydrate intakes and only allow consuming less than 30g daily!**

The standard ketogenic diet actually prescribes at least 5% of calories each day from carbohydrates. We may have different body compositions, so it could be possible that you may achieve your most efficient ketone levels by taking 20g of carbs daily while another individual may consume 40g to reach their optimal state of ketosis.

Nevertheless, 30 grams of carbohydrates per day is the rule of thumb in the keto world. You may wonder how or what a 30-gram of carbohydrate intake looks like. (The 80-recipes for breakfast, lunch, dinner, snacks, and desserts, as well as the different meal plans in this guidebook, will show you how and what).

You may even be afraid of eating leafy greens since you will be dodging carbohydrates like Neo dodging a spray of bullets in the Matrix. Thus, therein lays **the main predicate and purpose of this guidebook—to develop your will and intuition for taking only 30 grams of carbohydrates so you will be more comfortable consuming the nourishing whole foods you need while skipping the junk foods you do not.**

Carbohydrates per se are neither good nor bad. They are merely molecules where carbon bonds with water. However, fiber is a carbohydrate type that never influences blood glucose levels. In the first place, fiber is insoluble and goes through the body undigested. It is only essential for a healthy and normal gut function, where the gut bacteria in the large intestine break them down.

Hence, for a clearer picture of a 30-gram carb comprising whole foods with fiber, you just subtract the fiber from the total carbohydrate value. For instance, if a whole food contains 8 grams of carbs with 5 grams of fiber, you would net 3 grams of carbs.

Equally important is to be cautious with your protein consumptions. Ingesting substantial quantities of protein will cause your body to convert the protein excesses into glucose. Besides, heavy protein consumptions tend to increase insulin levels, which control the metabolism of carbohydrates. In effect, this hinders your goal of achieving optimal ketosis.

In resolving this dilemma of reverting into breaking down of carbohydrates, it would be highly advisable to satisfy your gastronomic cravings with more fats. Although this may sound queer, such a peculiar advice will certainly weave wonders for you!

In principle, consuming more fats allows you to feel fuller. It suppresses abruptly your appetite or curbs your intents of taking more food serving portions. As a result, your high fat regimen will ensure lesser protein and carbohydrate ingestions. In the process, it directly addresses your excessive weight issues. Certainly, your insulin levels drop and your body attains optimal ketosis.

To repeat, maximizing your results under a ketogenic dietary program is to attain the metabolic state of optimal ketosis. The trick is not only to restrict your intakes of carbohydrates but also to be fully aware of partaking proteins. The secret, unbelievably, is to have your fill of fats...lots of fats! Your only problem now is to know how much fats, proteins, and carbohydrates you should take to attain optimal ketosis.

Ketogenesis/Ketosis Macronutrient Model: Ideal Implementation of the Correct Caloric Configuration Consumption

There are six main groups of macronutrients: carbohydrates, proteins, fats, vitamins, minerals, and water. The majority of the daily diets nowadays involve consuming calories with about 50% of carbohydrates, 35% of fats, and 15% of proteins.

Oppositely, the ketogenic diet consists almost exclusively of fats and proteins (at a specific dose per kilogram of your ideal body weight). As previously mentioned, your objective is to draw your energy primarily from fats via ketones and secondarily from glucose reserves.

Therefore, as a standard macronutrient model for undergoing ketogenesis/ketosis, your total DAILY caloric configuration consumption should approximately be as follows:

🍖 **70% to 80% of calories from fats**

🍖 **15% to 25% of calories from proteins**

🍖 **5% to 10% of calories from carbohydrates**

These ketogenic macronutrient ratios are very important and you should always be aware of them. By this caloric configuration[7], it apparently translates to considering the following conditions for your body to reach ketosis:

🍖 **Consume enough fats.**

🍖 **Update the proteins in your food recipes and meal plans regularly.**

⦿ Minimize your carbohydrate consumption.

These conditions must always complement each other. They should not go as one without the other. If you consume fewer carbohydrates but also lesser fats, you will be feeling tired constantly and depriving your body of energy. Conversely, if you eat more fats and you do not alter your carbohydrate consumption, you will surely fail and gain more weight due to excess calorie intakes!

Due to this seeming caloric imbalance, it would be necessary to supplement the diet with additional sources of vitamins and minerals. Of course, you should maintain drinking the traditional 6 to 8 glasses of water daily.

Each of the rated caloric percentages helps you to derive your recommended daily calorie intake. You will then know what food to eat and how much of each macronutrient category you should consume based on your specific body composition and lifestyle.

Implementing strictly the ketogenic diet may baffle patients, caregivers, or practitioners alike with its seeming difficulties. This is chiefly due to your presumed time devoted to and spent in planning and measuring your keto meals.

Nonetheless, any unplanned meals will imminently lead to breaking the momentum of your regular requirements for a nutritional balance. Thus, for the regimen's optimum efficiency, always try to consume your measured foods! Always plan before you use! Always apply the keto ratios! Always conform to the keto values!

Keystone Labels for Ketone Levels: Knowing the Kismets of Ketosis

While you follow the standard macronutrient consumptions of a keto diet, you might be unable to know whether your body is in a state of ketosis. During the first week of practicing the keto diet, ketosis can cause unpleasant symptoms such as fatigue, headaches, bad breath (fruity smell), thirstiness, and weakness. Once your body becomes adaptive to it, it would be difficult for you to know whether your liver is actually producing ketone bodies to provide your body with the energy it needs.

Alternatively, you are unsure whether your body has an excess of ketone bodies. An overproduction of ketones promotes *ketoacidosis* (high acidity levels in your blood), which leads further to health complications. Thus, it is indeed important to check or measure your ketone levels.

Typically, ketone bodies manifest in your urine. You can apply the traditional spot test, which uses chemically coated dipsticks you can easily avail from your local pharmacy. If the analyzed urine contains *acetoacetic acid* (ketones), the reactive surface of the dipstick changes its color. The color chart printed on the package has labeled parameters, which allow you to compare the color and determine the approximate amount or concentration of ketone bodies in your urine.

However, dipsticks are generally unreliable since they do not render accurate measurements. They rather leave you clueless about the exact concentration levels and presence of ketones.

More innovative but pricey blood glucose measuring gadgets are more reliable to give you accurate measurements. While most of these devices require pricking your forefinger with a needle for a blood sample, you can readily determine the precise levels of your ketones within seconds.

The following will be your guidelines in interpreting the differently ranged values of ketone concentrations, measured in *mmol/L* (millimoles per liter):

➔ **Below 0.50-mmol/L** denotes a ketone count that is way beyond optimum levels of burning fat. Under this range, your body is not in a state of ketosis but only depicts to have normal levels of ketone bodies.

➔ **Within 0.50 to 1.50-mmol/L** signifies a moderate ketone count, which results in a better metabolism of fats and weight reduction with no deficiencies of insulin. However, this range does not indicate optimum conditions of ketosis. Instead, this only connotes that your body is undergoing a lighter or normal nutritional ketosis.

➔ **Within 1.50 to 3.0-mmol/L** portrays the recommended ketone levels for optimum weight loss. This specific range essentially exhibits the ideal values for attaining a state of optimum nutritional ketosis. Nonetheless, you should be on the lookout when reaching on the verge of a higher ketone level. In all likelihood, you will be at risk of incurring diabetic ketoacidosis. Consult immediately with your doc for further advice.

→ **Above 3.0-mmol/L** demonstrates achieving neither worse nor better conditions as compared to ketone levels within the 1.5o to 3.0 mmol/L range. Thus, the ketone counts within this range are often negligible values. However, higher ketone levels only imply that your body is either having lesser food intakes or having a serious metabolic issue. For the latter, prompt medical care is necessary.

Just the same, it is never advisable to exceed 80 mg/dL (8-mmol/L) or a dark purple color on the dipstick. If this occurs to you, ask yourself if you have been drinking enough fluids; or better, increase your carbohydrate intake. If you clearly exceed this level, it may be a sign that your body has difficulties with the metabolism of ketones. This situation is very rare, but it requires an immediate examination by your doctor.

The ideal time to measure your ketones is during the beginning of the evening (because during the day, the amount of ketones in your urine is usually low). If you do it during the day, ensure having an empty stomach, or preferably, before breakfast.

Alternatively, choose a time when you are performing your usual daily tasks. Yet, never perform the test right after an intensive activity since your body cells will have a greater need for energy sourced from ketone bodies in your blood.

Actually, attaining the ideal metabolic state of optimum nutritional ketosis is achieving your healthy weight loss goals and wellness agenda. More importantly, it is reaping a host of the regimen's rewards.

Chapter 2-Reaping the Regimen's Remarkable Rewards

Despite the fact that the intended establishment of the ketogenic dietary program was initially for the treatment of seizures, epilepsy, and other issues of the nervous system, legions of individuals have now accepted to practice the regimen with a variety of reasons or goals. Foremost of these goals is to reap the regimen's remarkable reward for losing extra poundage while at the same time gaining more energy.

More significantly, the continued popular practice of the diet stems from a myriad of wellness benefits. For the record, the prestigious European Journal of Clinical Nutrition[8] compiled the following report in June 2013 about the following general health and wellness issues that the keto diet has been dealing with successfully:

♥ **Reducing Rapidly Weighty Weights**[9] – Cutting down on your carbohydrate intake is among the most effective, yet, simplest ways to reduce weight. Research even shows that people indulging in low-carbohydrate and high-fat diets tend to lose more weight quicker compared to most practitioners of low-fat diets (not to mention that low-fat dieters aggressively limit their calorie intakes)!

Aside from the fact that your body virtually becomes a fat-burning machine, the major reason behind this favorable rapid weight reduction outcome is that the keto diet decreases insulin levels. A low insulin level stimulates the appropriate retention of sodium contents in your body. Meaning, your body normally experiences a diuretic effect, inducing urination to drain the excess body fluids. In effect, your kidney starts to rid out excess sodium, which actually causes fluid retention or a temporary fluid weight gain.

♥ **Curbing Cravings and Abating Appetites**[10] – A regular intake of fats suppresses automatically your sweet tooth cravings, as well as your intents for extra servings. Hence, even if you do not try, you will frequently end up consuming only the ideal keto calorie amounts. With a healthier lifestyle that includes physical exercises, along with a declining level of your appetite, they complement the process of reducing your unwanted bulks and bulges!

♥ **Optimizing Optimistic Outlooks** – Since the diet prompts you to eat fats, your brain consequently sources its energy from the breaking down of fats. Studies, needless to say, show that fat metabolism results in lesser depression and stress symptoms, uplift overall moods, and more satisfaction and happiness in life.

♥ **Modifying Symptoms of the Metabolic Syndrome**[11] – Over the long term, ketosis helps to reduce the number of health risks and issues by altering or reversing the dreaded *metabolic syndrome*—an aggregation of the following dangerous symptoms:

- Low Levels of High-Density Lipoprotein (HDL)
- High Levels of Low-Density Lipoprotein (LDL)
- High Levels of Triglycerides (TG)
- High Blood Pressure Levels
- High Blood Sugar and Insulin Levels
- Obesity or Destructive Abdominal Fats Buildup

♥ **Qualifying Qualitative LDL & Quantitative HDL** – The main function of lipoproteins in your body is to convey fatty cholesterols in your bloodstreams. Your *'bad cholesterol'* or LDL transports fats from your liver to the different cells and organs of your body. Your *'good cholesterol'* or HDL carries fats from your body to your liver, which may excrete or reuse them as ketone bodies. For a diet rich in fats, your LDL levels decrease while your HDL levels increase.

In other words, high quantities of HDL enhance fat metabolism while degraded qualities of LDL restrict the circulation of bad cholesterols in your body. Being such the case, this gives rise to balanced cholesterol levels that will prevent incurring risks of various heart ailments and stroke.

♥ **Trimming and Taming Triglycerides (TG)** – A common indicator of acquiring CHD is incurring high TG-to-HDL ratios. In most cases, your blood triglyceride levels have tendencies of shooting up, especially when you indulge with a low-fat regimen.

Since the keto diet can increase your HDL levels through rich intakes of fats, it only follows that your TG-to-HDL ratios logically decrease. This also means that there will be a constant reduction of fat molecules in your bloodstream.

♥ **Hampering the Happenstance of Hypertension** – High blood pressure, also termed as *hypertension*, is a principal risk factor for many health issues such as CHD, stroke or decreased levels of oxygen in the brain, kidney failure, dementia or other neurodegenerative disorders, and several others. Medical research about the keto diet shows that blood pressure reductions are directly proportionate to reduced consumptions of sugary and starchy carbohydrates.

♥ **Disabling the Development of Diabetes**[11, 12] – A low-carbohydrate intake also results in decreased insulin and blood sugar levels. In short, it prevents the onset of prediabetes conditions, as well as Type-II diabetes mellitus.

Essentially, Type-II diabetes mellitus appears to characterize high blood sugar levels that your body cannot reduce on its own. The reason for your body's difficulty to lower blood sugar levels is commonly due to *insulin resistance*[13], whereby, your body can no longer produce sufficient insulin hormones to keep blood sugar levels down to their normal range.

♥ **Overcoming Obesity**[14] – The recommended macronutrient or caloric consumption values of the regimen result in controlling *insulin spikes* (secretion of insulin) and prevent drastic upswings in your blood sugar levels. Additionally, your regulated calorie intake destroys the accumulation of destructive stored fats in your abdominal cavity. Hence, aside from suppressing of your appetite, the diet prevents you to incur obesity issues while maintaining a healthy weight.

♥ **Curtailing Conceptions of Cancer Cells** –Similar to your body cells, a tumor cell produces energy. It flourishes by usually tapping glucose sourced from starchy carbohydrates to burn at extremely rapid rates compared to other cells in your body. They only weaken and ultimately cease to thrive with an abundance of fats around and a decreased glucose supply.

💙 **Boosting Brainpower & Cognitive Capabilities**[15] – With enhanced blood sugar and balanced cholesterol levels, you will gain optimum blood vessel health. This also indicates that your healthy blood vessels can constantly supply sufficient amounts of oxygen, as well as ketones to your brain cells to burn for energy. Compared to glucose, ketones can prevent your brain cells from undergoing destructive processes of *oxidative stress* (release of free radicals, which results in cellular degeneration), Hence, ketosis reduces your risks of acquiring Alzheimer's disease, Parkinson's disease, and other forms of neurodegenerative dysfunction or mental deterioration.

💙 **Leasing Longer Lives & Leading Lively Lifestyles** – As the keto diet secures a specific macronutrient requirement that provides your ideal daily calorie consumption for general healthcare, it also lowers your chances of developing symptoms of muscle weakness or frailty by about 70%. Thus, you can be as dynamic as you can be. Moreover, since the diet also lessens your risks of developing life-threatening illnesses, you virtually reduce your mortality risks by roughly 20% at any age!

Chapter 3- Starting & Sticking to the Program's Proper Performances

Fundamentally, the ketogenic dietary program is a holistic medical nutrition therapy. It involves crucially particular participants from the various medical disciplines.

Your entire medical team may include a neurologist/physician who has the vast experiences in prescribing the diet; a certified nurse who is knowledgeable enough about the cause and effects of the regimen; and, a professional dietitian who shall coordinate with the regular implementation of the dietary program.

In addition, more assistance and support may need the services of a licensed pharmacist who shall advise about the specific dosages of prescribed carbohydrate values and medicines, and perhaps, a registered medical social practitioner who shall collaborate with your family. Finally, for the safe and proper program performance, other medical caregivers, as well as your immediate family members should have the necessary understanding and information about the various important aspects of the regimen.

As you get to start practicing the keto dietary plan, always heed the wise advice of availing the guidance and close supervision of your medical adviser. Inevitably, there are somehow risks of complicating health matters during your initiation to the program aside from acquiring the keto flu and other side effects.

For instance, if you are suffering from Type-1 diabetes mellitus, you should forego proceeding to attain optimal ketosis since it can pose further harm to your health. Nevertheless, if ketone bodies are indeed present in your bloodstream, ensure that your blood sugar should be at normal levels.

Having a normal blood sugar level indicates that your body can be at normal ketosis, similar to the states of ketosis exhibited by healthy practitioners of a strict low-carbohydrate regimen. On the contrary, having a high blood sugar level with an abundance of ketones only denotes that insulin levels are extremely low.

Although non-diabetics do not typically suffer from these risky blood sugar levels, they may acquire *diabetes acidosis*, or ketoacidosis, which could be life-threatening. When such condition happens, your body requires more insulin injections.

However, prudence will dictate that you should seek medical advice, especially when you are not sure at all. Gaining higher ketone levels for the sake of losing weight will never be worth the risk for individuals with Type-1 diabetes mellitus.

Regimen's Requirements & Regulations

Practicing the keto diet may eventually take several forms. Thus, it is only prudent to repeat some significant details discussed previously to etch in mind and avoid confusion. **However, its standard practice remains to comprise a daily carbohydrate consumption of not more than 30 grams.**

As you keep your carbohydrates restricted, you will be inclined to consume often meals derived principally from fats, dairy, vegetables, and nuts. Specifically, your meals should be a composition of ample amounts of animal and vegetable fats, including proteins sourced from dairy produce, vegetables, and nuts.

More importantly, follow strictly the formulaic daily ketogenic nutritional value proportions of 70%-80% calories from fats, 15%-25% calories from proteins, and 5%-10% calories from carbohydrates! You should also bear in mind that a high-protein intake would prevent your body from reaching optimal nutritional ketosis. Thus, set your daily protein consumptions with respect to the percentage of your body fat and lean body mass. To calculate:

You first figure out the percentage of your body fat.

Your body fat percentage X your weight = your amount of fat.

Your lean body mass = your weight – your amount of fat.

The daily amount of your protein intake = 0.8 X your lean body mass, in pounds

If you prefer using metric units and calculations, then you multiply 1.8 by your lean body mass in kilograms.

Rationalizing Rated Ratios

The rated caloric ratios in a keto diet are alternative calculations for your required daily caloric consumptions. Oftentimes, these rated ratios are importantly applicable when taking into account the intensities of your daily activities.

The ketogenic diet uses the most common caloric ratios of 4:1 and 3:1. In details, a 4:1 ratio denotes a keto diet comprising 4 grams of fats for every gram of proteins including carbohydrates.

In short, for every 5 grams of consumed food, you will have 4 grams of fats and a gram of proteins/carbohydrates. Hence, a 4:1 keto diet consists of 80% fats (that is, 4÷5=80%) and 20% proteins/carbohydrates (that is, 1÷5=20%). Similarly, a 3:1 keto diet consists of 75% fats (that is, 3÷4=75%) and 25% proteins/carbohydrate (that is, 1÷4=25%).

As you will notice, the ketogenic rated ratios compare the quantities of fats, proteins, and carbohydrates expressed in grams, which is a weight measure. This is because you will be measuring your keto foods by their weight using a gram scale.

If you will compare fats, proteins, and carbohydrates in accordance to their provided number of calories instead of the provided number of grams, the concluding ratio would be slightly different. This stems from the fact that fats provide your body with more calories (9 calories per gram) compared to protein and carbohydrates (4 calories per gram).

For instance, you require consuming 360 calories. To provide your body with 360 calories from proteins/carbohydrates, you need to consume 90 grams of proteins/carbohydrates (that is, 360÷4=90). Yet, to receive the same number of calories from fats, you need to consume only 40 grams of fats (360÷9=40).

Fats actually provide your body with the same amount of calories with much lesser weight or mass since it is denser calorically compared to proteins and carbohydrates. Such being the case, the keto meals tend to appear smaller than those standard meals, despite providing exactly the same number of calories.

If you were on a 4:1 keto diet ratio, then that would mean a 90%-calorie in your diet comes from fat. Think again. Lest you confuse yourself further by wondering how it could be 80% fats and 90% fats at the same time, it is indeed 80% fat if you measure the diet by weight and 90% fat if you measure it by calories.

Put in mind that a 4:1 keto ratio signifies 4 grams of fat for every gram of proteins/carbohydrates. Thus, 4 grams of fat, which gives 9 calories per gram, provides a sum of 36 calories (that is, 4 x 9 = 36); 1 gram of proteins/carbohydrates, which gives 4 calories per gram, provides a sum of 4 calories (that is, 1 x 4 = 4). Alternatively, the calorie ratio of fat to proteins/carbohydrates is 36:4. This implies that each 40-calorie intake, 36 calories come from fat while 4 calories come from proteins/carbohydrates. Hence, 90% of the calories come from fat (that is, 36÷40=90%) while 10% come from proteins/carbohydrates (4÷40=10%).

Chapter 4-Grocery Guide

As you launch your keto dietary program but you are quite unsure where to take off and what foods to consume, the following food-shopping list comprises the most notable and recommended keto diet foods. The list, categorized under the major food groups is, by no means, extensive. Nonetheless, it directs you towards staying on course with your keto program.

Always remember to choose products rich in fats and low in carbohydrates when you are shopping for food items with your ketogenic diet. Fats are your source of energy!

However, always be careful! Read the product labels well. Labels of the different food products would surprise you to see how much sugar and carbs they contain!

In the beginning, you will have to work extra hard to find what you need, but you will get the hang of it over time. Like any other discipline or training, the keto regimen has its shares of difficulties at the start, especially when picking the right item from the grocery shelf. By practicing it with frequency, everything becomes easy as counting 123 and reciting ABC!

It would be a prudent advice though to stick to selecting and consuming mostly fresh and real foods. Real foods denote organic, unprocessed, and natural foods. Although processed or canned goods can be beneficial and convenient in a pinch, particularly when you wish on taking anything quickly with fewer carbohydrate contents, nothing beats consuming much healthier foods that are at their most natural form.

Inclusive Items for Constant Consumption (Recommended & Restricted Rations)

Basic Beverages
[Be cautious with drinks containing sweeteners since they may consist of carbohydrates.]
- Coffee *(with unsalted butter or cream, but no milk)*
- Carbonated or sparkling water
- Distilled water

Dairy Doses
[Preferably, opt for full fat, raw & organic dairy products. If you like to reduce weight, it is wise to skip all dairy items except for unsalted butter for your coffee.]
- All low-carb cheeses *(i.e., asiago, blue, brie, burrata, cheddar, Colby, cottage, cream, feta, Fontina, goat, gorgonzola, Gouda, Gruyere, Havarti, Manchego, Monterey Jack, mozzarella, Muenster, parmesan, pepper jack, provolone, ricotta, Romano, Roquefort, and Swiss)*
- Butter
- Clarified butter/ghee
- Cream
- Greek yogurt

Elemental Eggs
[Ideally, choose raw, organic, and free-ranged produces.]
- Chicken
- Duck
- Goose
- Pheasant
- Quail
- Turkey

Healthy Herbs & Spice Selections
[Herbs and spices, especially pre-made spices, are critical since they all contain many carbohydrates. Hence, note carefully their values in nutrition labels.]

Fresh Fruits
[Fruits are optional and are dependent on weight and health. While some cannot tolerate fructose, others remain slim and fit with it. Stick to typically low-fructose fresh fruits.]

- Avocado
- Berries
- Carambola/Starfruit
- Cherry
- Coconut
- Grapefruit
- Lemon/Lime
- Casaba melon
- Prickly pear
- Olives (black/green)

Favored Flours
[Since the ketogenic diet restricts all types of grains, only consider gluten-free or all other nut flours.]
- Almond
- Coconut
- Hazelnut
- Macadamia
- Pecan
- Walnut

Meaty Meals
[Enjoy liberally the fat and skin of grass-fed and organic meats.]
- Bacon *(if possible, charcuterie bacon with the least sugar and without nitrites/nitrates)*
- Biltong/jerky meat *(strips of sun-dried cured meat)*
- Cold cuts & delicatessen meats
- Cured meats *(with the least sugar content & without unknown curing agents and chemicals)*
- Game *(domestic/wild)*
- Livestock *(veal, pork, mutton, hogget & beef)*
- Offal *(internal parts)*
- Pemmican *(dried meat cuts mixed with melted fat)*
- Poultry
- Sausages *(with only meat & spices and without fillers/extenders like sugar, soya, rusk, rolled oats & gluten)*

Notable Nuts
[Avoid European chestnuts since they are steep with net carbs.]
- Almond
- Brazil
- Cashew
- Coconut
- Hazelnut
- Macadamia
- Peanut
- Pecan
- Pine

- Pistachio
- Sacha Inchi/Inca nut
- Walnut

Optimum Oils & Fundamental Fats
- Animal lard & fats
- Avocado oil
- Beef tallow
- Butter
- Coco cream/milk/oil
- Crème fraiche & other creams *(heavy, whipped & sour)*
- Macadamia oil
- Mayonnaise *(must be homemade, using the proper oils)*
- Nut butter
- Olive oil
- Schmaltz/duck fat

Pantry Picks
- Bouillon cubes/broth stocks *(i.e., vegetable, beef, pork, fish & chicken)*
- Canned/bottled low-carb vegetables *(i.e. beans, greens, pickles & sauerkraut, etc. with no added sugars)*
- Canned processed meats *(i.e., corned beef, luncheon meat, Vienna sausage, etc.)*
- Canned seafood *(i.e., anchovies, crab, salmon, sardines, shrimp & tuna)*
- Canned tomatoes *(juice, paste, sauce, dried or whole fruit)*
- Extracts *(vanilla, lemon, almond, etc., but avoid those with sugar)*
- Sauces & seasonings *(gluten-free and with no added sugars or thickeners)*
- Xanthan gum *(for binding & thickening)*

Seed Sources
- Chia
- Flaxseed/linseed
- Hemp
- Pumpkin
- Sesame
- Sunflower

Suited Sweeteners
[Use only sweeteners with low glycemic index (GI), which measures the amount of blood sugar raised by food. Use sparingly inulin, sucralose, tagatose, and xylitol. Skip aspartame, maltitol, monkfruit *(Luo Han Guo)*, saccharine, fructose syrup & high sugar alcohols.]
- Allulose
- Erythritol
- Stevia

Supported Seafood
[The keto diet supports global sustainable fishing practices; thus, as much as possible, fish and seafood should be under the list of Southern Africa Sustainable Seafood Initiative (SASSI).]
- Abalone
- Anchovy
- Angelfish *(Atlantic pomfret)*
- Calamari *(Cape Hod squid, baby calamari)*
- Crab *(fiddler, pea, oyster & soft-shell)*
- Dorado *(dolphinfish or mahi-mahi)*
- Eel *(kingklip, New Zealand, pink cusk)*
- Hake/cod
- Herring *(Atlantic, Baltic, redeye round)*
- Lobster *(East Coast rock)*
- Mackerel *(Atlantic, king, queen & Spanish)*
- Mussel *(black, blue, Chilean blue, Chinese, Mediterranean blue, green-lipped & white)*
- Oyster *(Pacific & Cape Rock)*
- Salmon *(blackfish, blueback, Cohoe, redfish, salmonid, sockeye,*
- Sardines
- Scallop *(Peruvian)*
- Seabream *(black bream, Hottentot, slinger)*
- Shrimps/prawns *(Kiddi, Indian)*
- Snoek *(barracuda)*
- Sprat *(Brisling sardine)*
- Squid *(Patagonian, Argentine shortfin, Cape Hope, European & Humboldt flying)*
- Stockfish *(shallow-water Cape Hake)*
- Trout *(rainbow)*
- Tilapia
- Tuna *(Albacore, yellowfin, skipjack)*
- Yellowtail

Veggie Viands
[Limit your choices to low-carb vegetables]
- Artichoke
- Asparagus
- Aubergine *(brinjal, eggplant, garden egg & mad apple)*
- Bell peppers
- Broccoli
- Bok choy
- Cabbage
- Carrot
- Cauliflower
- Celery
- Cucumber
- Garlic
- Green beans
- Kale
- Lettuce *(Batavian, Butterhead, buttercrunch, Chinese, cos or Romaine & loose-leaf)*
- Mushrooms
- Onions
- Pepper *(green)*
- Radish
- Shallots
- Snow/sugar snap peas
- Spinach
- Brussels sprouts
- Squash *(summer, spaghetti & vegetable marrow)*
- Swiss chard
- Tomato
- Zucchini

NOTE: When you consumed all the appropriate ketogenic food items, yet, you do not seem to shed off your excess weight, you must have been consuming too much proteins or dairy foods, nuts, and fruits. Thus, maintain your ideal keto macronutrient consumption.

Abbreviations

Measurements

c	cup
g	gram
kg	kilogram
l	liter
lb	pound
ml	milliliter
oz	ounce
pt	pint
tsp	teaspoon
tbsp	tablespoon

Special Diet Information

VEG	Vegetarian
V	Vegan
GF	Gluten-Free
DF	Dairy-Free
NF	Nut-Free

Chapter 5-Bountiful Breakfasts

1-Choco Chip Whey Waffles

Diet Specs: GF | VEG | DF

Yield: 4-waffles/2-servings

Serving Portion: 2-waffles

Preparation Time: 10 minutes

Cooking Time: 6 minutes

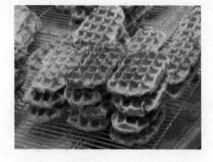

Ingredients:

2-tbsp organic coconut oil

2-tbsp coconut sugar

4-tbsp chocolate whey protein powder

⅓-cup almond flour

A pinch of salt

½-tsp baking powder

½-cup almond milk

2-pcs eggs

Directions:

1. Mix all the ingredients in the blender to obtain a homogenous paste.

2. Preheat your waffle iron. Pour the waffle dough in the iron and cook each waffle for 3 minutes.

Nutritional Values per Serving:

Calories: **423** | Fat: **32.8**g | Protein: **26.5**g | Total Carbohydrates: **8.3**g | Dietary Fiber: **2.9**g | Net Carbohydrates: **5.4**g

2-Coco Cinnamon-Packed Pancakes

Diet Specs: GF| VEG | NF | DF

Yield: 4-pancakes/2-servings

Serving Portion: 2-pancakes

Preparation Time: 30 minutes

Cooking Time: 5 minutes

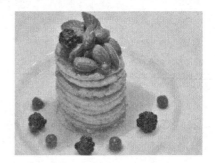

Ingredients:

2-pcs eggs

2½-tbsp organic coconut flour

¼-cup milk substitute with hydrogenated vegetable oil (or almond milk)

1-tbsp baking soda

½-tbsp cinnamon

½-tbsp baobab powder

2-tbsp organic coconut flower syrup

Directions:

1. In a salad bowl, mix the coconut flour, baobab powder, cinnamon, and baking soda.

2. Add the beaten eggs, the almond milk, and the coconut syrup. Let the dough rest for 30 minutes.

3. Cook the pancakes in a hot pan with coconut oil.

4. Dress the pancakes with raspberries/blueberries or almonds.

Nutritional Values per Serving:

Calories: **392** | Fat: **32.5**g | Protein: **20**g | Total Carbohydrates: **11.3**g | Dietary Fiber: **6.4**g | Net Carbohydrates: **4.9**g

3-Magdalena Muffins with Tart Tomatoes

Diet Specs: GF | VEG

Yield: 4-muffins/2-servings

Serving Portion: 2-muffins

Preparation Time: 10 minutes

Cooking Time: 20 minutes

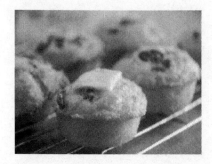

Ingredients:

2½-tbsp whole-wheat flour

2½-tbsp almond flour

1-tbsp yeast or baking soda

A dash of salt, pepper, and paprika

2-pcs eggs

1-tbsp organic cashew nuts

1-tbsp hemp oil

2½-tbsp soymilk

⅓-cup feta cheese, diced

1⅓-cup dried tomatoes, without oil and sliced into small pieces

Directions:

1. Mix the wheat flour, almond flour, yeast, and spices.

2. Then add eggs, cashews, oil, and soymilk.

3. Mix well to obtain a smooth paste. Add the feta and tomatoes.

4. Mix well and pour the dough into muffin pans previously greased with coconut oil.

5. Bake for 20 minutes at 350°F.

Nutritional Values per Serving:

Calories: **405** | Fat: **33.3**g | Protein: **20.3**g | Total Carbohydrates: **11**g | Dietary Fiber: **4.9**g | Net Carbohydrates: **6.1**g

4-Spinach Shoots Mediterranean Medley

Diet Specs: GF | VEG | NF

Yield: 2-servings

Serving Portion: 1 serving bowl

Preparation Time: 10 minutes

Cooking Time: 1 minute

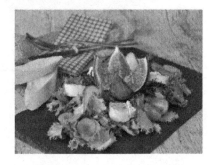

Ingredients:

½-cup spinach shoots

2-tbsp quinoa

¼-cup avocado, sliced

1-tbsp fresh goat cheese

1-tsp agave syrup, gluten-free

¼-cup dried blackberries

1-pc fig

1-tsp pumpkin seeds puree

Directions:

1. Arrange the spinach shoots, cooked quinoa, and avocado on a large plate.

2. Mix the goat cheese, agave syrup, and dried blackberries.

3. Make 4 small cuts in the fig so that you can open it and insert the goat cheese mixture.

4. Spread your fig on the spinach shoots. Sprinkle over with pumpkin seed puree.

Nutritional Values per Serving:

Calories: **308** | Fat: **26**g | Protein: **15.4**g | Total Carbohydrates: **9.7**g | Dietary Fiber: **6.5**g | Net Carbohydrates: **3.2**g

5-Romantic Raspberry Power Pancake

Diet Specs: GF | V | DF

Yield: 2-pancakes/one serving

Serving Portion: 2-pancakes

Preparation Time: 5 minutes

Cooking Time: 10 minutes

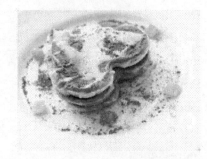

Ingredients:

2-tbsp raspberries, crushed

2-tsp almond flour

1-tbsp yeast or baking soda

1-tbsp vegan protein powder

2-tbsp soymilk

1-tbsp coconut oil

Directions:

1. Mix the crushed raspberries and dry ingredients.

2. Pour the milk and mix well to obtain a homogenous mixture.

3. Cook the pancakes for 2 minutes on each side using a little coconut oil in a pan. Flip the pancake when small bubbles appear.

4. Dress with almonds or nuts.

Nutritional Values per Serving:

Calories: **323** | Fat: **25.3**g | Protein: **15.7**g | Total Carbohydrates: **12**g | Dietary Fiber: **3.8**g | Net Carbohydrates: **4.8**g

6-Spinach Sausage Feta Frittata

Diet Specs: GF

Yield: 6-frittata wedges/6-servings

Serving Portion: 1-frittata wedge

Preparation Time: 15 minutes

Cooking Time: 30 minutes

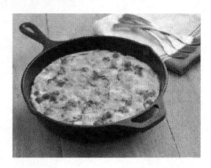

Ingredients:

10-oz. spinach, frozen, thawed, drained, and chopped

12-oz. sausage, sliced into small pieces

½-cup feta cheese, crumbled

½-cup almond milk, unsweetened

½-cup heavy cream

¼-tsp. ground nutmeg

½-tsp. salt

¼-tsp. black pepper

12-pcs eggs, whisked

Directions:

1. Place the sausage in a medium-sized mixing bowl. Break the spinach up into the same bowl as the sausage.

2. Sprinkle the cheese over the mixture. Toss lightly until fully combined. Lightly spread the mixture onto a greased 13" × 9" casserole dish, or greased muffin cups.

3. In a larger bowl, blend the almond milk, cream, nutmeg, salt, and pepper with the eggs, and mix well until fully combined.

4. Gently pour the mixture into the dish or muffin cups until for about ¾ full. Bake at 375°F for about 50 minutes (for the casserole), or 30 minutes (for the muffin cups), or until fully set.

Nutritional Values per Serving:

Calories: **295** | Fat: **22.9**g | Protein: **18.5**g | Total Carbohydrates: **4.6**g | Dietary Fiber: **1**g | Net Carbohydrates: **3.6**g

7-Mayonnaise Mixed with Energy Egg

Diet Specs: GF | VEG | NF

Yield: one serving

Serving Portion: 1 serving bowl

Preparation Time: 2 minutes

Cooking Time: 5 minutes

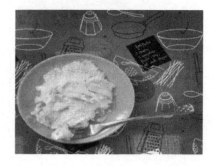

Ingredients:

2-tbsp organic mayonnaise, gluten-free

1-pc large egg

1-tbsp butter

Directions:

1. Mix the mayonnaise and egg in a medium-sized bowl until fully combined.

2. Melt the butter in a non-stick skillet. Pour the egg mixture, and cook until set. Scrape the egg and all remaining fat onto a serving plate. Serve immediately.

Nutritional Values per Serving:

Calories: **295** | Fat: **22.7**g | Protein: **18.8**g | Total Carbohydrates: **3.8**g | Dietary Fiber: **0.1**g | Net Carbohydrates: **3.7**g

8-Avocados atop Toasted Tartiné

Diet Specs: GF | VEG | NF

Yield: 2-tartinés/2-servings

Serving Portion: 1-tartiné

Preparation Time: 10 minutes

Cooking Time: 5 minutes

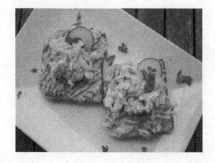

Ingredients:

2-slices bread, gluten-free

½-pc small avocado, thinly sliced

1-tbsp fresh cheese

1-tsp lemon juice

A dash of salt and pepper

1-tsp chia seeds for garnish (optional)

Directions:

1. Toast lightly the bread slices.

2. Carefully arrange the avocado slices on each bread slice. Drizzle with the lemon juice. Spread the fresh cheese. Sprinkle with a dash of salt and pepper. Top with garnish.

TIP: If you like a richer breakfast, you can serve this slice of bread with a slice of hard-boiled egg. You can also garnish the avocado toast with the watercress and chili flakes for a kick of early morning freshness.

Nutritional Values per Serving:

Calories: **268** | Fat: **22.4**g | Protein: **13.5**g | Total Carbohydrates: **8.9**g | Dietary Fiber: **6.7**g | Net Carbohydrates: **3.2**g

9-Fish Fillet & Perky Potato Cheese Combo

Diet Specs: GF | NF | DF

Yield: 2-servings

Serving Portion: 1 serving plate

Preparation Time: 15 minutes

Cooking Time: 10 minutes

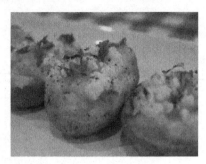

Ingredients:

1-tbsp olive oil

1-pc large potato, cooked and thinly sliced

¼-cup lean white cheese

½-tsp herbs of your choice

3.5-oz. herring fillet, steamed and sliced in half

½-tsp flaxseed oil or coconut oil

A dash of salt and pepper

Directions:

1. Heat a non-stick pan with olive oil. Add the potato slices and cook until browned.

2. Season the white cheese with salt, pepper, and herbs of your choice.

3. Arrange the potatoes equally between two plates. Top with the cheese and herring fillets. Garnish with a drizzle of flaxseed oil.

TIP: Fill in your sautéed potatoes with your favorite ingredients such as fresh onions, parsley or an egg.

Nutritional Values per Serving:

Calories: **298** | Fat: **24.9**g | Protein: **14.2**g | Total Carbohydrates: **6.5**g | Dietary Fiber: **3.2**g | Net Carbohydrates: **4.3**g

10-Cream Cheese Protein Pancake

Diet Specs: GF | VEG | NF

Yield: 4 x 6" diameter pancakes/2-servings

Serving Portion: 2-pancakes

Preparation Time: 10 minutes

Cooking Time: 12 minutes

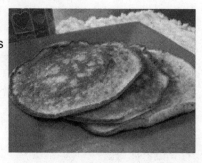

Ingredients:

2-pcs eggs

2-oz cream cheese

1-packet sweetener

½-tsp cinnamon

1-tbsp butter

Directions:

1. Combine all the ingredients except the butter in a blender. Blend until smooth. Let the batter stand for 2 minutes to allow the bubbles to settle.

2. Grease slightly a hot pan with ¼-tbsp butter. Pour ¼-batter into the pan. Cook for about 2 minutes until turning golden. Flip the pancake and cook for 1 minute on its other side.

3. Repeat the same cooking procedure with the remaining batter. Serve with fresh berries of choice and sugar-free syrup.

Nutritional Values per Serving:

Calories: **340** | Fat: **28.1**g | Protein: **16.2**g | Total Carbohydrates: **8.1**g | Dietary Fiber: **3.8**g | Net Carbohydrates: **4.3**g

11-Veggie Variety with Peanut Paste

Diet Specs: GF | VEG | DF

Yield: one serving

Serving Portion: 1 serving bowl

Preparation Time: 15 minutes

Cooking Time: 15 minutes

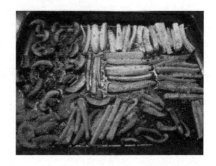

Ingredients:

1-bulb small onion, thinly sliced

¾-cup broccoli, sliced into quarters

1-pc small carrot, sliced into quarters

½-pc green pepper, thinly sliced

5-pcs mushrooms, sliced into quarters

A dash of salt, pepper, and powdered chili

2-tbsp peanut butter, dairy-free

2-tbsp. soy sauce, gluten-free

1-tbsp agave syrup (or honey), gluten-free

¼-cup red cabbage, thinly sliced

Directions:

1. Pour a little water in a heated skillet and cook the onions until they are transparent. Add the broccoli, carrot, pepper, and mushrooms. Cook for 10 minutes until tender. (Add a little water if the pan is too dry). Season the veggies with a dash of salt, pepper, and chili.

2. For the sauce, mix the peanut butter with the soy sauce, agave syrup, and 3 tbsp water.

3. To serve, incorporate the red cabbage. Garnish the dish with the sauce.

TIP: To lessen the calories, the dish uses water instead of oil. If you use oil, preferably coconut oil, you increase the calories by 100.

Nutritional Values per Serving:

Calories: **349** | Fat: **28.7**g | Protein: **18.4**g | Total Carbohydrates: **10.8**g | Dietary Fiber: **6.5**g | Net Carbohydrates: **4.3**g

12-Avocado Aliment with Egg Element

Diet Specs: GF | VEG | NF | DF

Yield: 2-servings

Serving Portion: 1-halved stuffed avocado

Preparation Time: 8 minutes

Cooking Time: 20 minutes

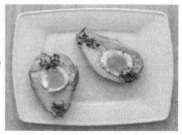

Ingredients:

1-pc egg, whisked

1-pc avocado, halved, pitted, and removed slightly with flesh

A dash of sea salt and pepper

1-tbsp parsley, chopped

1-tsp cayenne pepper

Directions:

1. Preheat your oven to 375°F.

2. Pour the egg gently into each halved avocado. Remove the excess liquid.

3. Place the stuffed avocado in a baking tray. Bake for 20 minutes.

4. Season the preparation with sea salt, parsley, and cayenne pepper.

Nutritional Values per Serving:

Calories: **275** | Fat: **23.8**g | Protein: **11.8**g | Total Carbohydrates: **10.7**g | Dietary Fiber: **4**g | Net Carbohydrates: **3.4**g

13-Pumpkin Pancakes

Diet Specs: GF | VEG | DF

Yield: 6-pancakes/3-servings

Serving Portion: 2-pancakes

Preparation Time: 10 minutes

Cooking Time: 30 minutes

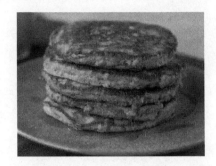

Ingredients:

1-tsp vanilla extract

1-cup coconut cream

3-pcs eggs

2-tbsp egg whites

½-cup pumpkin puree

5-packs sweetener

4-tbsp ground flax seed

4-tbsp ground hazelnuts or hazelnut flour

1-tsp yeast or baking powder

1-tbsp black tea powder

1-tbsp. coconut oil for cooking

Directions:

1. Whisk together the first five liquid ingredients for half a minute until they become frothy. Mix the dry ingredients in a separate bowl.

2. Combine both the dry and liquid ingredients to obtain a batter. (Add water, as necessary if the mixture is too thick.)

3. Grease a saucepan with a teaspoon of coconut oil. Ladle in the first pancake.

4. Cover the pan and cook for 3 minutes. Flip and cook the other side.

5. Repeat the cooking process until using up all the batter.

Nutritional Values per Serving:

Calories: **200** | Fat: **16.4**g | Protein: **11**g | Total Carbohydrates: **5.2**g |
Dietary Fiber: **3**g | Net Carbohydrates: **2.2**g

14-Whole-Wheat Plain Pancakes

Diet Specs: VEG | NF | DF

Yield: 2-pancakes/1-serving

Serving Portion: 2-pancakes

Preparation Time: 5 minutes

Cooking Time: 12 minutes

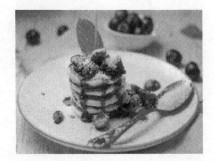

Ingredients:

2-pcs eggs

4-tbsp whole-wheat flour

½-tsp yeast or baking soda

⅓-cup sunflower oil

1-tbsp coconut oil for cooking

Directions:

1. Mix all the ingredients in a bowl until obtaining a smooth consistency.

2. Pour the coconut oil in a pan placed over medium heat. Cook for 3 minutes until browned. Flip and cook the other side.

3. Serve hot and garnish with fresh fruits of your choice such as blueberries, strawberries or raspberries, nuts, and coconut flakes.

TIP: You can mix some blueberries in the batter to create delicious blueberries pancakes.

Nutritional Values per Serving:

Calories: **329** | Fat: **27.6**g | Protein: **16.1**g | Total Carbohydrates: **5.4**g | Dietary Fiber: **1.3**g | Net Carbohydrates: **4.4**g

15-Blueberries Breakfast Bowl

Diet Specs: GF | V | NF | DF

Yield: one serving

Serving Portion: 1 serving bowl

Preparation Time: 35 minutes

Cooking Time: 0 minutes

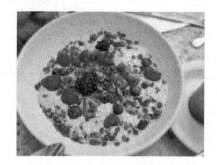

Ingredients:

1-tsp chia seeds

1-cup almond milk

¼-cup fresh blueberries or fresh fruits

1-pack sweetener for taste

Directions:

1. Mix the chia seeds with the almond milk. Stir periodically.

2. Place in the fridge to cool for 30 minutes, and then serve with fresh fruit. Enjoy!

TIP: For an even better taste, let it sit in the fridge for a night and add fresh fruits in the morning.

Nutritional Values per Serving:

Calories: **202** | Fat: **16.8**g | Protein: **10.2**g | Total Carbohydrates: **9.8**g | Dietary Fiber: **5.8**g | Net Carbohydrates: **2.6**g

16-Feta-Filled Tomato-Topped Oldie Omelet

Diet Specs: GF | VEG | NF

Yield: one serving

Serving Portion: 1 omelet

Preparation Time: 5 minutes

Cooking Time: 6 minutes

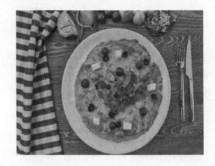

Ingredients:

1-tbsp coconut oil

2-pcs eggs

1½-tbsp milk

A dash of salt and pepper

¼-cup tomatoes, sliced into cubes

2-tbsp feta cheese, crumbled

Directions:

1. Beat the eggs with the milk, salt, pepper, and the remaining spices.

2. Pour the mixture into a heated pan with coconut oil.

3. Stir in the tomatoes and cheese. Cook for 6 minutes or until the cheese melts.

TIP: Add your favorite spices to the omelet for more fun.

Nutritional Values per Serving:

Calories: **335** | Fat: **28.4**g | Protein: **16.2**g | Total Carbohydrates: **4.5**g | Dietary Fiber: **0.8**g | Net Carbohydrates: **3.7**g

17-Ave Avocado Super Smoothie

Diet Specs: GF | VEG

Yield: one serving

Serving Portion: 1 serving bowl

Preparation Time: 10 minutes

Cooking Time: 1 minute

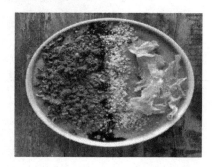

Ingredients:

½-cup Greek yogurt

7-oz. frozen avocados

½-cup water

½-tsp vanilla powder

1-tsp each chia seeds, chocolate chips, and peanut butter for garnish

Directions:

1. Mix all the ingredients. You can also crush them in the blender.

2. Pour the smoothie into a bowl and garnish to your taste with fruits, seeds or nuts.

Nutritional Values per Serving:

Calories: **398** | Fat: **33.1**g | Protein: **20**g | Total Carbohydrates: **15.5**g | Dietary Fiber: **10.6**g | Net Carbohydrates: **4.9**g

18-Hearty Hodgepodge

Diet Specs: GF | NF | DF

Yield: one serving

Serving Portion: 1 serving bowl

Preparation Time: 5 minutes

Cooking Time: 25 minute

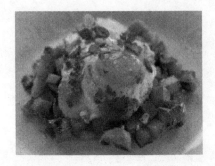

Ingredients:

1-bulb small onion, diced

1-tbsp coconut oil

1-tbsp bacon bits

1-pc medium zucchini, diced into squares

1-tbsp parsley or chives, chopped

¼-tsp. of salt

1-pc large egg, fried

Directions:

1. Sauté the onion with coconut oil in a pan placed over medium heat. Add the bacon, stirring frequently until both onion and bacon turn slightly brown.

2. Add the zucchini, and cook for 15 minutes. Remove from heat and transfer the preparation in a serving bowl. Sprinkle over the parsley.

3. To serve, top the dish with the fried egg.

Nutritional Values per Serving:

Calories: **290** | Fat: **24**g | Protein: **14.6**g | Total Carbohydrates: **6.7**g | Dietary Fiber: **3.1**g | Net Carbohydrates: **3.6**g

19-Chocolate Chia Plain Pudding

Diet Specs: GF | VEG | NF

Yield: 3-servings

Serving Portion: 1 serving bowl

Preparation Time: 55 minutes

Cooking Time: 0 minutes

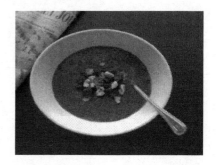

Ingredients:

3-tbsp chia seeds

2-cups water

¼-cup whey chocolate protein

½-cup Greek yogurt, sugar-free

¼-cup linseeds, roasted

1-tbsp cocoa powder, unsweetened

1-packet sweetener (optional)

Directions:

1. Mix the chia seeds with water and let stand for 20 minutes. Stir occasionally.

2. Once the chia seeds are well inflated, add all the other ingredients and mix again.

3. Place in the fridge for 30 minutes before serving.

TIP: Serve with raspberries or blueberries. For a vegan variant, it is possible to use a vegetable yogurt and chocolate vegetable protein.

Nutritional Values per Serving:

Calories: **370** | Fat: **28.7**g | Protein: **22.3**g | Total Carbohydrates: **10.8**g | Dietary Fiber: **5.2**g | Net Carbohydrates: **5.6**g

20-Seasoned Sardines with Sunny Side

Diet Specs: GF | NF | DF

Yield: one serving

Serving Portion: 1 serving bowl

Preparation Time: 5 minutes

Cooking Time: 10 minutes

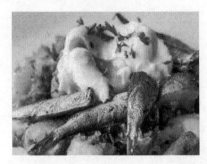

Ingredients:

2-oz. sardines in olive oil

2-pcs eggs

½-cup arugula

¼-cup artichoke hearts, diced

A pinch of salt

A dash of black pepper

Directions:

1. Preheat your oven to 375°F.

2. Place the sardines in an oven-ready stoneware bowl. Add the eggs on top of the sardines. Top the eggs with the arugula and artichokes. Sprinkle with salt and pepper.

3. Bake for 10 minutes until the eggs cook through.

Nutritional Values per Serving:

Calories: **255** | Fat: **21**g | Protein: **13.5**g | Total Carbohydrates: **4.9**g | Dietary Fiber: **1.8**g | Net Carbohydrates: **3.1**g

Chapter 6-Luscious Lunch

1-Pulled Pepper-Lemon Loins

Diet Specs: GF | NF | DF

Yield: 4-servings

Serving Portion: 1 chicken loin

Preparation Time: 15 minutes

Cooking Time: 360 minutes

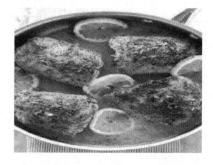

Ingredients

½-stick of butter

1-pc large lemon, sliced

1-pc green pepper, chopped

1-tbsp garlic, minced

2-tbsp olive oil

1-tbsp salt

1-tsp dried thyme

½-tbsp Dijon mustard

3-lbs. (4-pcs) chicken tenderloins

1-cheddar cheese slice, shredded

4-leaves romaine lettuce

Directions:

1. Combine the butter, lemon, pepper, garlic, oil, salt, thyme, and mustard in your slow cooker. Switch the slow cooker on high and melt the butter.

2. Add the chicken; ensure to coat the chicken with the butter mixture.

3. Cook on low for 6 hours or on high for 4 hours. Add the cheese and let it sit for 15 minutes on low.

4. To serve, place the chicken over a bed of lettuce leaves.

Calories: 280 | Fat: 23.3g | Protein: 14g | Total Carbs: 4.1g | Dietary Fiber: 0.6g | Net Carbs: 3.5g

Nutritional Values per Serving:

Calories: **280** | Fat: **23.3**g | Protein: **14**g | Total Carbohydrates: **4.1**g | Dietary Fiber: **0.6**g | Net Carbohydrates: **3.5**g

2-Shrimps & Spinach Spaghetti

Diet Specs: GF | NF | DF

Yield: 2-servings

Serving Portion: 1 serving plate

Preparation Time: 5 minutes

Cooking Time: 8 minutes

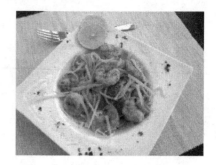

Ingredients:

8-tbsp vegetable broth

1-cup low carb spaghetti, rinsed and drained

1-pc leek, cut into strips

1⅓-cup frozen peas

1⅓-cup fresh spinach leaves

¼-lb. shrimp, pre-cooked

1-tbsp lemon zest

1-pc green pepper, finely chopped (divided, per serving)

2-pcs basil leaves (divided, per serving)

1-pc lemon (divided, per serving)

Directions:

1. Pour the vegetable broth in a wok and cook for 5 minutes. Add the leeks, peas, spinach, and shrimp. Cook further for 5 minutes.

2. Add the spaghetti, and continue cooking for 2 minutes. Remove quickly from heat and pour into a bowl, mix with lemon zest.

3. Divide the pasta equally between two plates. To serve, garnish with the pepper, basil leaves, and lemon.

Nutritional Values per Serving:

Calories: **425** | Fat: **33**g | Protein: **25**g | Total Carbohydrates: **15.7**g | Dietary Fiber: **10.4**g | Net Carbohydrates: **5.3**g

3-Single Skillet Seafood-Filled Frittata

Diet Specs: GF | NF | DF

Yield: 4-frittata wedges/4-servings

Serving Portion: 1 frittata wedge

Preparation Time: 2 minutes

Cooking Time: 18 minutes

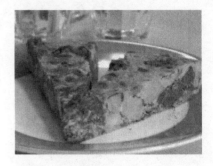

Ingredients:

1-pc green pepper

¼-pc lime, squeezed for juice

1-tbsp coconut flour

1-tbsp sesame oil

1-tbsp soy sauce, gluten-free

1-tbsp coconut oil

3-bulbs fresh onions, chopped

½-clove garlic, minced

¼-cup prawns, raw

1⅓-cup mussels, deshelled

2-pcs eggs, whisked

Directions:

1. Preheat your oven to 475°F. Meanwhile, make the sauce by combining the first five ingredients in a mixing bowl. Mix thoroughly until fully combined. Set aside.

2. Melt the coconut oil in a small skillet and fry the onions. Add the garlic, prawns, and mussels. Cook for 10 minutes until the prawns turn pink.

3. Stir in the eggs. Place the skillet in the oven and bake for 5 minutes.

4. Slice the frittata in four slices and serve with the sauce.

Nutritional Values per Serving:

Calories: **459** | Fat: **38.2**g | Protein: **22.9**g | Total Carbohydrates: **8.7**g | Dietary Fiber: **3**g | Net Carbohydrates: **5.7**g

4-Poultry Pâté & Creamy Crackers

Diet Specs: GF | NF

Yield: one serving

Serving Portion: 3-crackers topped with pate

Preparation Time: 15 minutes

Cooking Time: 35 minutes

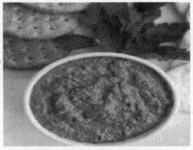

Ingredients:

3.5-oz. chicken livers

3-tbsp butter, softened

1-tsp. Italian seasoning

A pinch of salt and pepper

3-pcs unsalted creamy crackers, gluten-free

Directions:

1. Place all the ingredients in a blender except the crackers. Blend to a smooth paste consistency.

2. Serve with the crackers.

TIP: Instead of crackers, you can use radish slices.

Nutritional Values per Serving:

Calories: **437** | Fat: **36.4**g | Protein: **21.9**g | Total Carbohydrates: **5.5**g | Dietary Fiber: **0**g | Net Carbohydrates: **5.5**g

5-Chickpeas Carrots Curry

Diet Specs: GF | VEG | NF

Yield: one serving

Serving Portion: 1 serving bowl

Preparation Time: 5 minutes

Cooking Time: 25 minutes

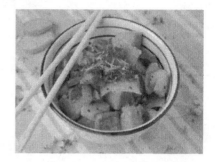

Ingredients:

½-bulb onion, finely chopped

½-pc carrot, sliced into cubes

½-tsp coconut oil

¼-cup chickpeas

½-tsp tomato paste

3-tbsp light soy cream

½-tsp turmeric powder

⅛-bunch fresh coriander

A pinch of salt, pepper, and sweet paprika

Directions:

1. Sauté the onions and carrots for 5 minutes with coconut oil in a skillet.

2. Add the chickpeas, tomato paste, soy cream, turmeric, coriander, and spices. Mix well and cook for 10 minutes.

3. Cook the rice for 10 minutes in boiling water. Serve the konjac rice with the vegetable curry and chickpeas.

Nutritional Values per Serving:

Calories: **380** | Fat: **30.9**g | Protein: **18**g | Total Carbohydrates: **14.4**g | Dietary Fiber: **10.7**g | Net Carbohydrates: **3.7**g

6-Baked Broccoli in Olive Oil

Diet Specs: GF | VEG | NF

Yield: 3-servings

Serving Portion: 1 serving bowl

Preparation Time: 5 minutes

Cooking Time: 25 minutes

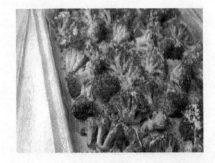

Ingredients:

1½-lbs broccoli florets

¼-cup olive oil

3-tsps garlic, minced

2-tbsp fresh basil, chopped

½-tsp red chili flakes

¾-tsp kosher salt

Zest of ½-pc lemon

Juice of ½-pc lemon

⅓-cup parmesan cheese

Directions:

1. Preheat your oven to 425°F.

2. Arrange the broccoli florets in a baking sheet lined with parchment paper.

3. Season the broccoli with olive oil, chopped fresh basil, minced garlic, kosher salt, red chili flakes, zest and juice of half a lemon each.

4. Sprinkle parmesan cheese over the broccoli. Place the sheet in the oven to bake for about 25 minutes.

Nutritional Values per Serving:

Calories: **484** | Fat: **39.2**g | Protein: **26.7**g | Total Carbohydrates: **21.6**g | Dietary Fiber: **16.8**g | Net Carbohydrates: **4.8**g

7-Bunless Bacon Burger

Diet Specs: GF | NF

Yield: 4-burgers/4-servings

Serving Portion: 1-bacon burger

Preparation Time: 8 minutes

Cooking Time: 37 minutes

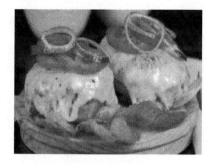

Ingredients:

1½-lbs. ground beef

2-tbsp olive oil

2-tbsp bacon bits

4-oz. pepper jack cheese

1-bulb onion, sliced crosswise

8-leaves romaine lettuce

A dash of salt and pepper

Directions:

1. Form the ground beef into four patties. Cook for 4 minutes with olive oil on a skillet placed over medium heat. Flip the patties to cook the other sides. Set aside.

2. Using the same skillet, stir-fry the bacon bits for 5 minutes until crispy.

3. Use the lettuce leaves as buns. Place each patty on a leaf and top with the bacon bits. Sprinkle a dash of salt and pepper. Top each burger with the cheese to melt.

Nutritional Values per Serving:

Calories: **435** | Fat: **36.3**g | Protein: **21.7**g | Total Carbohydrates: **6.1**g | Dietary Fiber: **0.7**g | Net Carbohydrates: **5.4**g

8-Smoky Sage Sausage

Diet Specs: GF | NF | DF

Yield: 4-patties/4-servings

Serving Portion: 1-patty

Preparation Time: 5 minutes

Cooking Time: 8 minutes

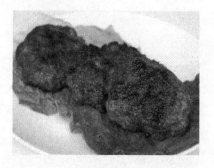

Ingredients:

2-tbsp sage, chopped

2-packets sweetener

1-tsp salt

1-tsp maple extract

1-lb. ground pork

½-tsp black pepper

¼-tsp garlic powder

⅛-tsp cayenne pepper

Directions:

1. Combine all the ingredients in a large mixing bowl.

2. Form patties from the mixture.

3. Put the patties in a skillet placed over medium heat. Cook for 4 minutes until cooked through. Flip the patties to cook on the other side.

Nutritional Values per Serving:

Calories: **170** | Fat: **13.2**g | Protein: **8.4**g | Total Carbohydrates: **5.3**g | Dietary Fiber: **1**g | Net Carbohydrates: **4.3**g

9-Steamed Salmon & Salad Bento Box

Diet Specs: GF | NF

Yield: 2-bento boxes

Serving Portion: 1 bento box

Preparation Time: 10 minutes

Cooking Time: 0 minutes

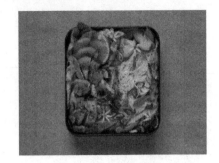

Ingredients:

2-pcs salad heads

1-cup carrot, grated

¼-cup cucumber, sliced

1-pc green pepper, thinly sliced

4-cups marinara pasta, rinsed, drained, and cooked for 2 minutes in boiling water

½-lb. salmon, steamed

2-pcs lemons

2-pcs eggs, boiled and sliced

1-tsp chia seeds

4-tbsp yogurt, sugar-free

1-tsp turmeric powder

½-pc lemon, zest

2-tbsp mint, minced

A pinch of pepper

Directions:

1. Divide equally the first eight ingredients between two bento boxes. Sprinkle the arrangements with chia seeds.

2. Mix the rest of the ingredients to make the sauce. Pack the sauce separately.

TIP: Tofu or minced meat is an option for fish while cucumber noodles are for pasta.

Nutritional Values per Serving:

Calories: **391** | Fat: **30.4**g | Protein: **24.9**g | Total Carbohydrates: **11.8**g | Dietary Fiber: **7.3**g | Net Carbohydrates: **4.5**g

10-Stuffed Spaghetti Squash

Diet Specs: GF | NF

Yield: 2-servings

Serving Portion: 1-halved stuffed squash

Preparation Time: 30 minutes

Cooking Time: 30 minutes

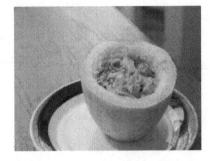

Ingredients:

1-pc spaghetti squash, halved and pitted

1-tsp olive oil

½-cup bacon strips, grilled

3-cups ground beef

1-pc green pepper, thinly sliced

½-bulb onion, sliced into cubes

1-tsp garlic powder

1-tsp paprika

A pinch of salt and pepper

1-cup cheddar cheese, grated

Directions:

1. Rub the squash halves with oil, and bake for 30 minutes at 350°F.

2. Meanwhile, roast the bacon in a saucepan placed over high heat. Stir in the onion and pepper. Add the beef and spices. Season the mixture with salt and pepper, and cook for 15 minutes, stirring regularly. Set aside.

3. Remove the flesh of the cooked squash by scratching with a fork. Mix the flesh with the meat mixture. Add the cheese, and put the mixture in the frayed squash.

4. Return the stuffed squash to the hot oven, and bake for 10 minutes.

TIP: The skin of the squash is thin and hard, so feel free to scrape deep to get the most flesh. You can use avocado instead of squash.

Nutritional Values per Serving:

Calories: **404** | Fat: **33.2**g | Protein: **20.3**g | Total Carbohydrates: **7**g |
Dietary Fiber: **1**g | Net Carbohydrates: **6**g

11-Prawn Pasta

Diet Specs: GF | NF | DF

Yield: 3-servings

Serving Portion: 1 serving plate

Preparation Time: 10 minutes

Cooking Time: 12 minutes

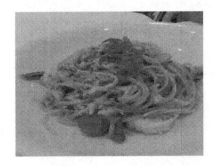

Ingredients:

1-tsp sesame seeds

1-pc lime

½-pc green pepper, thinly sliced

2 tbsp coconut flour

2-tbsp sesame oil

1-tbsp soy sauce, gluten-free

2-heads small cabbages

6-bulbs small onions, chopped

1-cup prawns, steamed

3-cups low-carb pasta, rinsed, drained, and cooked for 2 minutes in boiling water

8-pcs small radishes, sliced into 4-pieces for garnish

½-pc avocado, sliced for garnish

Directions:

1. Combine the first six ingredients in a bowl to make the pasta sauce. Set aside.

2. Cook the cabbage for 10 minutes in a pan with a little water and soy sauce. Add the onions and prawns. Cook for 2 minutes.

3. Arrange the pasta in a plate, topped with the prawn mixture, pasta sauce, and the garnishing.

TIP: You can replace shrimp with feta and sesame seeds with chia seeds.

Nutritional Values per Serving:

Calories: **393** | Fat: **32.8**g | Protein: **19.7**g | Total Carbohydrates: **14.9**g |
Dietary Fiber: **10.1**g | Net Carbohydrates: **4.8**g

12- Tasty Tofu Carrots &Cauliflower Cereal

Diet Specs: GF | VEG | NF | DF

Yield: one serving

Serving Portion: 1 serving bowl

Preparation Time: 20 minutes

Cooking Time: 20 minutes

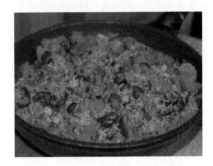

Ingredients:

For the Tofu-Carrots Mix:

½-block extra firm tofu, crumbled

2-tbsp reduced sodium soy sauce, gluten-free

½-cup onion, diced

1-cup carrot, diced

1-tsp turmeric

For the Cauliflower Cereal:

3-cups riced cauliflower

2-tbsp reduced sodium soy sauce, gluten-free

1½-tsp toasted sesame oil

1-tbsp rice vinegar

1-tbsp ginger, minced

½-cup broccoli, finely chopped

2-cloves garlic, minced

½-cup frozen peas

Directions:

1. Toss the tofu with the rest of the tofu-carrots mix ingredients. Place the mixture in your air fryer basket. Lock the lid, and set to cook for 10 minutes at 370°F.

2. Meanwhile, toss together all of the cauliflower cereal ingredients. Add this mixture to the air fryer pan. Lock the lid, and set to cook for another 10 minutes at 375°F.

Nutritional Values per Serving:

Calories: **390** | Fat: **32.6**g | Protein: **19.5**g | Total Carbohydrates: **17.4**g | Dietary Fiber: **12.7**g | Net Carbohydrates: **4.7**g

13-Stuffed Straw Mushroom Mobcap

Diet Specs: GF | VEG | NF

Yield: one serving

Serving Portion: 1-cup stuffed mushroom

Preparation Time: 15 minutes

Cooking Time: 5 minutes

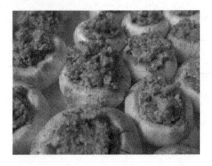

Ingredients:

1-cup fresh spinach, washed, bathed in ice, and drained

1-cup straw mushrooms or Chinese mushroom, washed and stems removed

1-tbsp coconut oil

1-bulb onion, finely chopped

1-clove garlic, minced

A dash of salt and pepper

A pinch of nutmeg

¼-cup quinoa, cooked

3.5-oz. cottage cheese

Directions:

1. Spread the spinach leaves over the food film while rolling them.

2. Fry the mushrooms with coconut oil in a saucepan before adding onion and garlic. Season the mushrooms with salt, pepper, and nutmeg. Set aside.

3. Combine the cooked quinoa with the cottage cheese. Spread the mixture evenly on the spinach leaves then roll into a pudding with the help of the food film.

4. Stuff the mushroom heads with the spinach pudding, and place them in the fridge.

5. Just before serving, slice the mushroom head with a sharp knife and pass quickly to the pan to heat.

Nutritional Values per Serving:

Calories: **401** | Fat: **34.7**g | Protein: **17.2**g | Total Carbohydrates: **16.9**g | Dietary Fiber: **11.4**g | Net Carbohydrates: **5**g

14-Crispy Chicken Packed in Pandan

Diet Specs: GF | NF | DF

Yield: 4-servings

Serving Portion: 1 chicken thigh

Preparation Time: 30 minutes

Cooking Time: 18 minutes

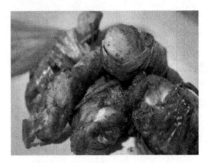

Ingredients:

4-pcs (½-lb.) chicken thigh

1-tbsp shallot

1-pc lemon

1-tsp of fennel seeds

1-tsp of turmeric powder

1-tsp of chili powder

1-tbsp of oyster sauce, gluten-free

A pinch of salt

A pinch of sugar

A handful of pandan leaves

Directions:

1. Preheat your air fryer to 350°F for about 5 minutes.

2. Marinate the chicken with all the ingredients. Set aside for 30 minutes.

3. Wrap each chicken meat with the pandan leaves.

4. Arrange the wrapped chicken in the air fryer basket and lock the lid

5. Set to cook for 18 minutes at 375°F.

Nutritional Values per Serving:

Calories: **382** | Fat: **32.5**g | Protein: **17.8**g | Total Carbohydrates: **7.7**g | Dietary Fiber: **3.1**g | Net Carbohydrates: **4.6**g

15-Chicken Curry Masala Mix

Diet Specs: GF | NF | DF

Yield: 3-servings

Serving Portion: 1 serving bowl

Preparation Time: 10 minutes

Cooking Time: 35 minutes

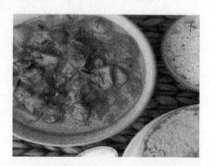

Ingredients:

2-tbsp sesame oil (divided)

2-tbsp ginger, diced

1½-lbs chicken thighs, boneless, skinless, and diced

1-cup tomatoes, chopped

¼-cup coriander, chopped

2-tsp turmeric

1-tsp cumin

1-tsp cayenne

2-tbsp lemon juice

Cilantro or mint leaves for garnish

Directions;

1. Sauté the ginger and jalapeno pepper with half of the sesame oil in a saucepan. Add the. Stir in the chicken, tomatoes, and coriander. Add the spices, the remaining sesame oil, lemon juice and half a cup of water.

2. Cover the saucepan, and cook for 30 minutes.

3. To serve, pour everything in a deep salad bowl, and garnish with cilantro or mint leaves.

Nutritional Values per Serving:

Calories: **377** | Fat: **29.3**g | Protein: **23.4**g | Total Carbohydrates: **6.8**g | Dietary Fiber: **1.9**g | Net Carbohydrates: **4.9**g

16-Milano Meatballs with Tangy Tomato

Diet Specs: GF | NF

Yield: 6-meatballs/3-servings

Serving Portion: 2 meatballs

Preparation Time: 25 minutes

Cooking Time: 30 minutes

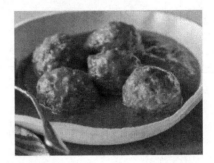

Ingredients:

For the Meatballs:

1-lb extra-lean ground beef

1-pc egg, whisked

10-pcs sun-dried tomatoes, chopped

½-cup ricotta cheese

1-cup Parmigiano-Reggiano cheese or parmesan cheese, freshly grated

A pinch of salt and freshly ground black pepper

For the Tomato Sauce:

1-bulb onion, finely chopped

¼-cup extra-virgin olive oil

2-lbs. tomato puree, gluten-free

A pinch of salt and freshly ground black pepper

Directions:

1. Combine all the meatball ingredients in a mixing bowl. Mix well until fully combined. Form balls from the mixture, and pat them down for even cooking.

2. Sauté the onions with olive oil in a skillet until they are translucent. Add the tomato puree and bring to a boil. Add the remaining ingredients and the meatballs. Cook for 30 minutes on medium heat.

TIP: For a vegetarian version of this recipe, you may replace the beef and pork meat with avocado and red potatoes.

Nutritional Values per Serving:

Calories: **396** | Fat: **32.6**g | Protein: **20.9**g | Total Carbohydrates: **8.2**g | Dietary Fiber: **3.4**g | Net Carbohydrates: **4.8**g

17-Aubergine À la Lasagna Lunch

Diet Specs: GF | VEG | NF

Yield: 2-lasagna sets/4-slices

Serving Portion: 1 lasagna slice

Preparation Time: 20 minutes

Cooking Time: 30 minutes

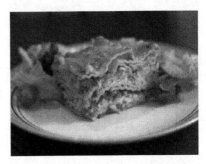

Ingredients:

2-pcs large eggplants, sliced and drained from excess liquid with a paper towel

A pinch of sea salt

2-cups part-skim ricotta cheese

½-cup parmesan cheese, freshly grated

1-pc egg, whisked

4-cups homemade tomato sauce, sugar-free

2-tbsp part-skim mozzarella cheese, shredded

2-tbsp cheddar cheese, grated

2-tbsp parsley, chopped

Directions:

1. Preheat your oven to 375°F. Meanwhile, season the eggplant slices with salt. Grill the eggplant slices for 3 minutes on each side.

2. Combine the ricotta, parmesan, and egg in a large bowl. Set aside.

3. Spread half of the tomato sauce in a saucepan. Layer half of the eggplant slices, and top with half of the cheddar and mozzarella. Pour half of the ricotta mixture over the layer, or just enough to coat it.

4. Cover the saucepan and insert into your preheated oven. Bake for 25 minutes. Set to cool for 10 minutes.

5. Repeat the process for the second lasagna set. To serve, garnish your lasagna with chopped parsley

Nutritional Values per Serving:

Calories: **346** | Fat: **27**g | Protein: **21.4**g | Total Carbohydrates: **7.9**g |
Dietary Fiber: **3.5**g | Net Carbohydrates: **4.4**g

18-Beef Broccoli with Sesame Sauce

Diet Specs: GF | NF | DF

Yield: 4-servings

Serving Portion: 1 serving bowl

Preparation Time: 10 minutes

Cooking Time: 45 minutes

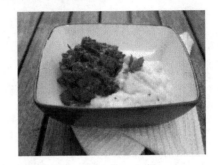

Ingredients:

2-tbsp coconut oil

1-tsp arrowroot powder

1-tbsp sesame oil

1-tbsp red fish sauce

½-tsp light sea salt

¼-tsp black pepper

¼-tsp baking powder

1-lb. beef, sliced into ¼-inch thick chunks

2-tsp sesame oil or olive oil

1-head broccoli, diced

2-tbsp coconut oil

2-cloves garlic, minced

2-ginger, finely chopped

A pinch of salt and pepper

Directions:

1. Mix the first seven ingredients in a bowl to make the sesame sauce. Set aside.

2. Fry the meat with sesame oil for 15 minutes until browned.

3. In a saucepan with water, add the broccoli, oil, garlic, and ginger. Season it with a pinch of salt and pepper. Add and spread the fried beef with the broccoli. Cover and cook for 20 minutes. Pour the sauce and cook for 10 more minutes.

Nutritional Values per Serving:

Calories: **375** | Fat: **31**g | Protein: **19.5**g | Total Carbohydrates: **5.4**g | Dietary Fiber: **0.8**g | Net Carbohydrates: **4.6**g

19- Sautéed Sirloin Steak in Sour Sauce

Diet Specs: NF

Yield: 4-servings

Serving Portion: 1 serving bowl

Preparation Time: 10 minutes

Cooking Time: 30 minutes

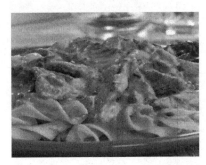

Ingredients:

1-bulb medium onion, chopped

1-clove garlic, minced

2-tbsp butter

1-lb. sirloin steak, trimmed and cut into thin strips

½-tsp salt

¼-tsp pepper

1-tbsp thyme

1½ cup fresh mushrooms, sliced

1-tbsp red wine vinegar

1-(10.5 oz.) can cream of mushroom soup

2-tbsp sour cream

4-cups egg noodles, cooked according to package instructions

Directions:

1. Sauté the onion and garlic with melted butter in a large skillet placed over medium heat. Remove from pan and set aside.

2. Add the beef strips, salt, pepper, and thyme. Cook evenly over low heat until browned.

3. Return the onion and garlic, and stir in the mushrooms, wine vinegar, and soup. Cover and simmer for 7 minutes until mushrooms are tender. Uncover and add sour cream. Stir and heat through. Serve immediately over the prepared noodles.

Nutritional Values per Serving:

Calories: **350** | Fat: **29.3**g | Protein: **17.7**g | Total Carbohydrates: **4.9**g | Dietary Fiber: **1**g | Net Carbohydrates: **3.9**g

20-Flaky Fillets with Garden Greens

Diet Specs: GF | NF | DF

Yield: 4-servings

Serving Portion: 1-fish fillet

Preparation Time: 25 minutes

Cooking Time: 30 minutes

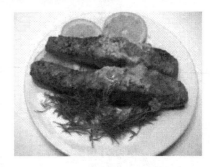

Ingredients:

1-lb broccoli, chopped into cubes and seasoned with a dash of salt and pepper

2-tbsp coconut oil

7-pcs scallions

2-tbsp small capers

1-tbsp sesame oil or olive oil

1½-lbs. white fish, sliced into 4 fillets

1-tbsp dried parsley

1¼-cups whipping cream, gluten-free and sugar-free

1-tbsp mustard, sugar-free

1-tsp of salt

¼-tsp ground black pepper

⅓-cup olive oil

5-oz.leafy greens

Directions:

1. Sauté the seasoned broccoli with sesame oil in a pan, and add the scallions and capers. Add the fish in the middle of the sautéed greens. Simmer for 15 minutes.

2. Meanwhile, mix the parsley with the whipping cream and mustard. Pour it over the cooked fish and vegetables. Drizzle with a little bit of coconut oil.

3. Return the saucepan on medium heat and cook for an extra 10 minutes.

Nutritional Values per Serving:

Calories: **395** | Fat: **33**g | Protein: **19.8**g | Total Carbohydrates: **8.7**g | Dietary Fiber: **3.9**g | Net Carbohydrates: **4.8**g

Chapter 7-Dinner Delights

1-Pizza Pie with Cheesy Cauliflower Crust

Diet Specs: GF | VEG | NF

Yield: 4-pizza wedges/2-servings

Serving Portion: 2-pizza wedges

Preparation Time: 5 minutes

Cooking Time: 30 minutes

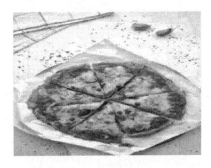

Ingredients:

½-head cauliflower, rinsed, riced, cooked for 5 minutes in boiling water, and drained

2-pcs eggs, whisked

⅓-parmesan cheese

½-cup cherry tomatoes, washed and halved

2-tbsp organic hempseed oil

1-tsp balsamic vinegar

1-mozzarella cheese ball, crumbled

¼-cup basil leaves

Directions:

1. Spin the cooked cauliflower in a dishtowel to let out as much liquid as possible. (The goal is to obtain a flour texture.) Add the eggs and cheese. Mix well.

2. Spread to a disk the cauliflower dough on a baking pan lined with parchment paper. Bake for 15 minutes at 400°F in your preheated oven.

3. Meanwhile, mix the tomatoes with hempseed oil and balsamic vinegar. Season the mixture with salt and pepper.

4. Remove the pizza dough from the oven. Add the tomato mixture and sprinkle over with mozzarella. Return the pan in the oven and bake further for 15 minutes.

5. Serve hot and garnish with fresh basil leaves.

Nutritional Values per Serving:

Calories: **384** | Fat: **32.1**g | Protein: **19.9**g | Total Carbohydrates: **5.5**g |
Dietary Fiber: **1.7**g | Net Carbohydrates: **3.8**g

2-Roasted Rib-eye Skillet Steak

Diet Specs: GF | NF

Yield: 2-servings

Serving Portion: 1 slice rib-eye steak

Preparation Time: 5 minutes

Cooking Time: 15 minutes

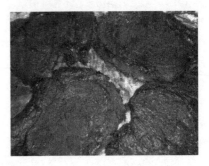

Ingredients:

1-16oz rib-eye steak (1 to 1¼-inch thick)

2-tbsp duck fat or peanut oil (divided)

A dash of salt and pepper

1-tbsp butter

½-tsp thyme, chopped

Directions:

1. Preheat your oven to 400°F. Place a cast iron skillet inside.

2. Season the rib-eye steak with oil, salt, and pepper.

3. Take the preheated skillet out from the oven and place over the stove, set in medium heat. Pour oil, and add the steak. Sear for 2 minutes on both sides.

4. Return the skillet with the steak in the oven. Roast for 6 minutes.

5. Remove the skillet and place over the stove, set in low heat. Add the butter and thyme in the skillet. Baste the steak for about 4 minutes.

Nutritional Values per Serving:

Calories: **722** | Fat: **60.2g** | Protein: **45g** | Total Carbohydrates: **0g** | Dietary Fiber: **0g** | Net Carbohydrates: **0g**

3-À la Spaghetti with Asian Sauce

Diet Specs: GF | VEG | DF

Yield: 2-servings

Serving Portion: 1 serving plate

Preparation Time: 10 minutes

Cooking Time: 15 minutes

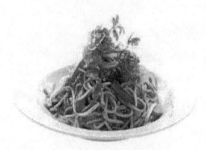

Ingredients:

For the Sauce:

2-tbsp soy sauce, gluten-free

1-tsp of hemp oil

1-tsp of lemon juice

1-tbsp peanut butter

For the Spaghetti:

½-bulb onion, diced

1-tsp coconut oil

1-tsp red or green pepper, diced

1-pc carrot, thinly sliced lengthwise

1 egg, whisked

5-oz. low-carb spaghetti, rinsed and cooked for 2 minutes in boiling water

Fresh coriander and peanuts for garnish

Directions:

1. Combine all the sauce ingredients in a bowl. Set aside.

2. Sauté the onion with oil, and add the peppers, carrots, egg, sauce, and spaghetti. Cook for 13 minutes, stirring frequently.

3. To serve, garnish with fresh coriander and peanuts.

Nutritional Values per Serving:

Calories: **412** | Fat: **34.4**g | Protein: **20.9**g | Total Carbohydrates: **10.5**g | Dietary Fiber: **5.7**g | Net Carbohydrates: **4.8**g

4-Shirataki & Soy Sprouts Pad Thai with Peanut Tidbits

Diet Specs: GF | VEG | DF

Yield: one serving

Serving Portion: 1 serving bowl

Preparation Time: 10 minutes

Cooking Time: 5 minutes

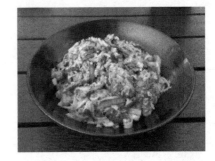

Ingredients:

For the Sauce:

1-tbsp peanut butter

2-tbsp soy sauce, gluten-free

½-lime

2-tbsp agave syrup, gluten-free

½-tbsp organic turmeric

For the Noodles:

1-bag of konjac shirataki noodles, rinsed and cooked for 2 minutes in boiling water

1-pc carrot, thinly sliced

1-bulb onion, thinly sliced

½-cup soy sprouts

¼-cup unsalted peanuts

Some sprigs of fresh coriander

Directions:

1. Combine all the sauce ingredients in a bowl. Set aside.

2. Heat the pasta with a little coconut oil in a frying pan. Pour the sauce and add the coriander. Mix well and cook for 5 minutes.

3. To serve, place in a bowl and garnish with peanuts and coriander sprigs.

Nutritional Values per Serving:

Calories: **423** | Fat: **35.2**g | Protein: **21**g | Total Carbohydrates: **14.9**g |
Dietary Fiber: **9.6**g | Net Carbohydrates: **5.3**g

5-Charred Chicken with Squash Seed Sauce

Diet Specs: NF | DF

Yield: 2-chicken skewers/one serving

Serving Portion: 2-chicken skewers

Preparation Time: 15 minutes

Cooking Time: 20 minutes

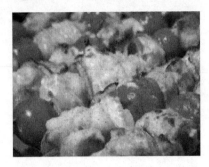

Ingredients:

For the Sauce:

2-tbsp white almond puree

2-cloves of garlic, finely chopped (divided, for the sauce and chicken marinade)

½-tbsp squash seeds

1-tbsp barley

1-pc fresh basil

For the Marinade:

2-branches rosemary, finely chopped

1-pc red chili, finely chopped

1-pc lemon (keep the zest)

Pinch of salt and ground black pepper

1-tbsp olive oil

1-cup chicken breasts, cubed

5-bulbs small onions, sliced in quarters

5-pcs cherry tomatoes

Directions:

1. Combine and mix all the sauce ingredients in a bowl. Set aside.

2. Mix all the marinade ingredients and let stand for 10 minutes. Thread alternately the onions, meat, and tomatoes into the skewers and grill over coal fire for 10 minutes on each side. Serve the chicken kebabs with the squash seed sauce.

Nutritional Values per Serving:

Calories: **428** | Fat: **35.6**g | Protein: **21**g | Total Carbohydrates: **16.9**g | Dietary Fiber: **11.6**g | Net Carbohydrates: **5.3**g

6-Therapeutic Turmeric & Shirataki Soup

Diet Specs: NF | DF

Yield: one serving

Serving Portion: 1 serving bowl

Preparation Time: 10 minutes

Cooking Time: 32 minutes

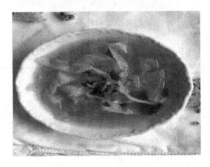

Ingredients:

1-tbsp turmeric powder

1-serving chicken-vegetable broth soup

3-pcs carrots, sliced into small pieces

3-slices ginger

1-pack (5-oz.) konjac shirataki noodles

¼-lb. chicken breast, sliced into strips

Directions:

1. Simmer all the ingredients over low heat for 30 minutes.

2. Rinse the konjac noodles thoroughly under cold water.

3. Add the noodles to the broth and heat for 2 minutes.

TIP: This is a great therapeutic dish when acquiring keto flu.

Nutritional Values per Serving:

Calories: **415** | Fat: **34.6**g | Protein: **21.6**g | Total Carbohydrates: **10.1**g | Dietary Fiber: **5.7**g | Net Carbohydrates: **4.4**g

7-Fresh Fettuccine with Pumpkin Pesto

Diet Specs: VEG | NF

Yield: 3-servings

Serving Portion: 1 serving bowl

Preparation Time: 15 minutes

Cooking Time: 2 minutes

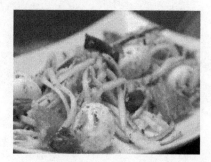

Ingredients:

For the Pesto Sauce:

1-tbsp olive oil

1-tbsp pumpkin seed oil

½-tsp pumpkin seeds

¼-cup barley

1-tbsp lemon juice

A pinch salt

For the Pasta:

1¾-cup zucchini, washed, peeled, and cut into thin noodle strips

½-cup cherry tomatoes, washed and cut in half

1¼-cup low carb fettuccine

1-pc mozzarella cheeseball

A pinch of pepper

Directions:

1. Combine and mix all the sauce ingredients with 2-tbsp water in a bowl. Set aside.

2. Boil the fettuccine for 1 minute and add the zucchini. Boil further for another minute, and drain.

3. Toss the pasta with the pesto sauce. Season the dish with a pinch of pepper and garnish with tomatoes and mozzarella.

Nutritional Values per Serving:

Calories: **417** | Fat: **34.7**g | Protein: **20.9**g | Total Carbohydrates: **10.5**g | Dietary Fiber: **5.3**g | Net Carbohydrates: **5.2**g

8- Cheddar Chicken Casserole

Diet Specs: GF | NF

Yield: 6-servings

Serving Portion: 1 serving plate

Preparation Time: 10 minutes

Cooking Time: 30 minutes

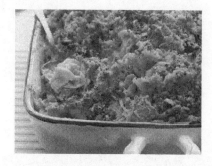

Ingredients:

20-oz. chicken breasts

2-tbsp olive oil (divided)

2-cups broccoli, steamed

½-cup sour cream

½-cup heavy cream

1-oz. pork rinds, crushed

A dash of salt and pepper

½-tsp paprika

1-tsp oregano

1-cup cheddar cheese, grated

Directions:

1. Preheat your oven to 450°F.

2. Sear the chicken with a tablespoon of olive oil in a pan until it cooks all the way through. Shred the meat in the pan. Add the remaining oil, broccoli, and sour cream.

3. Place and spread evenly the mixture in an 8" x11" pan. Press firmly and drizzle with heavy cream. Add all the remaining seasonings and top the casserole with the cheese. Place the pan in the oven and bake for 25 minutes until the edges turn brown and start bubbling.

Nutritional Values per Serving:

Calories: **405** | Fat: **33.8**g | Protein: **22.7**g | Total Carbohydrates: **3.6**g | Dietary Fiber: **1**g | Net Carbohydrates: **2.6**g

9-Zesty Zucchini Pseudo Pasta & Sweet Spanish Onions Overload

Diet Specs: VEG | NF | DF

Yield: 2-servings

Serving Portion: 1 serving bowl

Preparation Time: 10 minutes

Cooking Time: 20 minutes

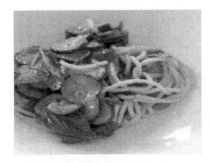

Ingredients:

2-tbsp of vegetable oil

2-pcs yellow onions or Spanish onions

1-tbsp low-sodium soy sauce

2-tbsp low-sodium teriyaki sauce

1-tbsp sesame seeds

4-pcs small zucchinis, sliced into spaghetti strips using a spiral cutter

Directions:

1. Add the vegetable oil, onions, and soy sauce to a saucepan placed over medium heat. Stir in the teriyaki sauce and sesame seeds. Mix well until fully combined.

2. Cook for 10 minutes, stirring frequently until the vegetables turn brown.

3. Add the zucchini pasta and cook for 3 minutes.

4. To serve, transfer the pasta in a serving dish and garnish with chopped parsley.

Nutritional Values per Serving:

Calories: **319** | Fat: **25.9**g | Protein: **18.1**g | Total Carbohydrates: **6.6**g | Dietary Fiber: **3.2**g | Net Carbohydrates: **3.4**g

10-Soba & Spinach Sprouts

Diet Specs: GF | VEG | DF

Yield: 2-servings

Serving Portion: 1 serving bowl

Preparation Time: 15 minutes

Cooking Time: 0 minutes

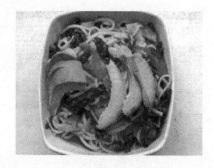

Ingredients:

3-pcs mushrooms, sliced into quarters

⅓-cup smoked tofu, sliced into squares

1-tbsp coconut oil

½-pc green pepper, sliced into strips

3-tbsp cashew nuts

½- clove garlic

½-pc lime, juice

A dash of salt and pepper

¼-cup water (more, as needed)

¼-cup soba noodles, cooked according to package instructions

1⅓-cup spinach sprouts

1-tbsp coconut shavings for garnish

Directions:

1. Fry the mushrooms and tofu with coconut oil in a frying pan until they turn brown. Add the pepper. Set aside.

2. For the sauce, mix cashews with garlic, lime juice, salt, pepper, and a little water.

3. Divide the noodles between two bowls and top with spinach sprouts. Arrange the remaining vegetables on top. Garnish with coconut shavings or avocado slices, sesame seeds, and a slice of lime.

4. To serve, pour over the sauce on each arranged bowl.

Nutritional Values per Serving:

Calories: **355** | Fat: **29.6**g | Protein: **17.8**g | Total Carbohydrates: **8.3**g | Dietary Fiber: **3.9**g | Net Carbohydrates: **4.4**g

11-Chickpeas & Carrot Consommé

Diet Specs: GF | VEG | NF | DF

Yield: 2-servings

Serving Portion: 1 serving bowl

Preparation Time: 10 minutes

Cooking Time: 20 minutes

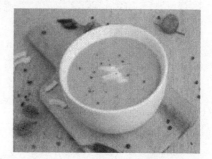

Ingredients:

¼-lb. chickpeas, cooked

1-tbsp coconut oil

1-clove garlic, minced

1-piece ginger, minced

1-bulb small onion, finely chopped

½-lb. carrots, sliced into small pieces

1¼-cup vegetable broth

A dash of salt and pepper

½-cup coconut milk

1-tbsp coconut shaving

Directions:

1. Arrange the chickpeas on a plate lined with parchment paper. Sprinkle with salt, curry, and paprika. Spread the spices well and bake for 15 minutes at 350°F.

2. Melt the coconut oil in a saucepan and brown the garlic, ginger, and onion. Add the carrots. Deglaze with vegetable broth and simmer for 15 minutes over medium heat until the carrots cook through.

3. Season to taste with salt, pepper, curry, and paprika. Pour the coconut milk.

4. Mix the soup and garnish with chickpeas and coconut shavings.

TIP: This soup will also be delicious with sweet potatoes, potatoes, parsnip, beetroot, spinach, mushrooms, broccoli, peas, tofu, chicken, coriander or parsley.

Nutritional Values per Serving:

Calories: **460** | Fat: **38.2**g | Protein: **23.3**g | Total Carbohydrates: **10.1**g | Dietary Fiber: **4.3**g | Net Carbohydrates: **5.8**g

12-Chicken Cauliflower Curry

Diet Specs: GF | NF | DF

Yield: 2-servings

Serving Portion: 1 serving bowl

Preparation Time: 15 minutes

Cooking Time: 30 minutes

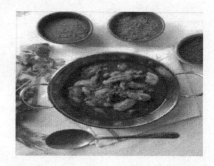

Ingredients

1-cup vegetable broth

1-tbsp curry paste

½-cup light coconut milk

½-lb chicken breast, cooked and sliced into small pieces

1-pc potato, diced

1-clove garlic, minced

½-bulb onion, finely chopped

1-cup cauliflower, diced

⅓-cup fresh peas

Salt and pepper

¼-cup goji berries

Directions:

1. Heat the vegetable broth in a wok for 5 minutes. Add the curry paste, coconut milk, meat, potato, garlic, and onion. Cook for 15 minutes.

2. Add the vegetables and cook further for 10 minutes until they are tender. Season the curry with a dash of salt and pepper.

3. To serve, garnish with goji berries.

TIP: If the sauce reduces too quickly, it is possible to add broth.

Nutritional Values per Serving:

Calories: **334** | Fat: **27**g | Protein: **18.7**g | Total Carbohydrates: **8.4**g | Dietary Fiber: **4.3**g | Net Carbohydrates: **4.1**g

13-Cheesy Cauliflower Mac Munchies

Diet Specs: GF | VEG

Yield: 2-servings

Serving Portion: 1 serving bowl

Preparation Time: 20 minutes

Cooking Time: 15 minutes

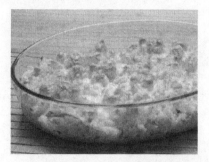

Ingredients:

1-pc medium cauliflower, riced

3-tbsp + ½-tsp avocado oil (divided)

A pinch of sea salt

A pinch of black pepper

1-cup cheddar cheese, shredded

¼-cup cream, gluten-free

¼-cup almond milk, unsweetened

Directions:

1. Preheat your air fryer to 400°F. Spray the pan with oil.

2. Place the riced cauliflower in the pan and drizzle with the avocado oil. Toss well and season with a pinch each of salt and pepper. Set aside.

3. Heat the cheese, cream, and milk with a little bit of avocado oil in a pot.

4. Pour the cheese mixture over the seasoned cauliflower. Lock the lid of the air fryer and set to cook for 14 minutes.

Nutritional Values per Serving:

Calories: **352** | Fat: **27.8**g | Protein: **20.9**g | Total Carbohydrates: **8.9**g | Dietary Fiber: **4.3**g | Net Carbohydrates: **4.6**g

14-Sugar Snap Pea Pods with Coco Crunch

Diet Specs: GF | VEG | NF | DF

Yield: 2-servings

Serving Portion: 1 serving bowl

Preparation Time: 5 minutes

Cooking Time: 10 minutes

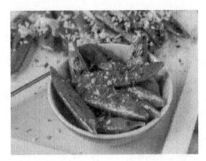

Ingredients:

4-tbsp salted butter, gluten-free and dairy-free

1-tbsp coconut oil

½-cup coconut, unsweetened and shredded

⅛-tsp cinnamon

1-tbsp rosemary oil

9-oz. snap pea pods, trimmed, strings removed, and diced

A pinch of salt

Directions:

1. In a saucepan, melt the coconut oil with the butter over medium heat. Add the coconut shreds, rosemary oil, and cinnamon. Toss very well until fully incorporated.

2. Add the diced pea pods and mix again. Leave to cook for 8 minutes until the pea pods start to melt.

3. To serve, sprinkle over a pinch of salt.

Nutritional Values per Serving:

Calories: **389** | Fat: **31.3**g | Protein: **22**g | Total Carbohydrates: **7.2**g | Dietary Fiber: **2.3**g | Net Carbohydrates: **4.9**g

15-Spicy & Smoky Spinach-Set Fish Fillets

Diet Specs: GF | NF | DF

Yield: 2-servings

Serving Portion: 1-fish fillet

Preparation Time: 15 minutes

Cooking Time: 10 minutes

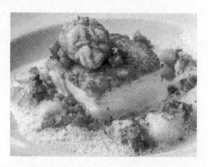

Ingredients:

2-pcs halibut meat (11-oz. each), membrane removed and deboned

4-cups packed spinach

Juice of ½-pc lemon

A pinch of salt and pepper

A pinch of smoked paprika

1-pc sliced lemon

1-pc green onions, sliced

1-pc red chili, deseeded and thinly sliced

1-cup cherry tomatoes, halved

2-tbsp avocado oil

Directions:

1. Place the halibut meat over a flat surface. Divide the spinach between them.

2. Lay each halibut meat on each pile of spinach. Squeeze the lemon over each part and season with smoked paprika.

3. Top each fish meat with lemon slices, green onions, chili, and the cherry tomatoes. Pour 1-tbsp of avocado oil over each fish portion.

4. Wrap around each fish meat tightly with foil; arrange them in a baking pan. Cook for 10 mins until the fish turns golden and flaky when forked.

TIP: You can use sesame or coconut oil instead of avocado oil and use salmon instead of halibut.

Nutritional Values per Serving:

Calories: **248** | Fat: **18.8**g | Protein: **15.3**g | Total Carbohydrates: **13.2**g | Dietary Fiber: **8.9**g | Net Carbohydrates: **4.3**g

16-Spicy Shrimps & Sweet Shishito

Diet Specs: GF | NF | DF

Yield: 2-servings

Serving Portion: 1 serving bowl

Preparation Time: 15 minutes

Cooking Time: 15 minutes

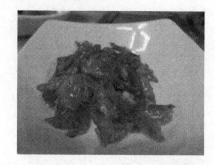

Ingredients:

2-tbsp canola oil

A pinch of sea salt

1-clove garlic, crushed and finely chopped

1-pc red chili pepper, seeded and finely chopped

5-oz. whole shishito peppers

10-oz. shrimps, jumbo size

1-tsp sesame oil

2-tbsp low-sodium light soy sauce

Juice of 1-pc lime

Directions:

1. Preheat your air fryer to 350°F for about 5 minutes. Spray your air fryer pan with canola oil.

2. Add the salt, garlic, and red chili pepper. Mix well until fully combined.

3. Add the shishito peppers; mix thoroughly again. Add the shrimps and drizzle with sesame oil.

4. Place the pan in your air fryer and lock the lid. Cook for about 10 minutes at 400°F

5. Divide the dish equally between three serving bowls. To serve, season each bowl with lime juice and soy sauce.

Nutritional Values per Serving:

Calories: **370** | Fat: **28.9**g | Protein: **23**g | Total Carbohydrates: **7.2**g | Dietary Fiber: **2.8**g | Net Carbohydrates: **4.4**g

17-Spaghetti-Styled Zesty Zucchini with Guacamole Garnish

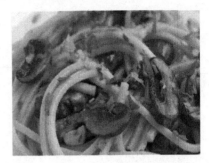

Diet Specs: GF | VEG | NF | DF

Yield: 2-servings

Serving Portion: 1-set of guacamole and carbonara

Preparation Time: 15 minutes

Cooking Time: 5 minutes

Ingredients:

2-pcs medium zucchini, cut into spaghetti strips using a spiral cutter

1-tbsp sea salt

1-pc large avocado, peeled, pitted, and cut into small pieces

1⅓-cup fresh basil, washed, dried and finely chopped

2-tbsp lemon juice

A dash of salt and black pepper

1-tbsp coconut oil

7-oz. mushrooms, cleaned and cut into slices

1-pc pomegranate, seeds extracted

Directions:

1. Season the zucchini strips with sea salt and set aside.

2. Mix the avocado slices, lemon juice, and a dash of salt and pepper. Set aside.

3. Toss lightly the zucchini in a frying pan placed over medium heat. Fry for 4 to 5 minutes in coconut oil. Add the mushrooms and pomegranate seeds.

4. To serve, place the zucchini spaghetti on a plate with the avocado cream in a separate bowl. Garnish with the basil leaves.

TIP: To peel quickly and cleanly a pomegranate, cut the fruit in half, and hold a half over a bowl or plate. Gently tap the back of the fruit with a tablespoon so that the beans come out. Scrape the most persistent grains directly with the spoon.

Nutritional Values per Serving:

Calories: **381** | Fat: **31.8**g | Protein: **19**g | Total Carbohydrates: **14.3**g | Dietary Fiber: **9.5**g | Net Carbohydrates: **4.8**g

18-Grain-less Gnocchi in Melted Mozzarella

Diet Specs: GF | VEG | NF

Yield: one serving

Serving Portion: 1 serving bowl

Preparation Time: 10 minutes

Cooking Time: 15 minutes

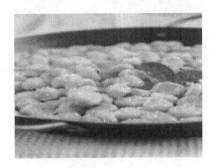

Ingredients:

2-cups mozzarella, shredded

½-tsp garlic powder

1-tsp salt

3-pcs large egg yolks, whisked (divided)

½-cup tomato sauce, gluten-free

Directions:

1. Melt the mozzarella with the garlic powder and salt for 5 minutes in a microwave-safe dish.

2. Pour half of the egg yolks into the mozzarella mixture in a large bowl. Mix until fully combined. Add the remaining egg yolks. Mix thoroughly again until fully incorporated.

3. Divide the mixture into four parts. Roll each part into a long rope over a flat surface. Cut each rope into gnocchi-like pieces, pressing each with a fork.

4. Bring a pan filled with water to a boil. Add the gnocchi dumplings and cook for about 2 minutes.

5. Preheat your air fryer to 350°F. Spray the air fryer pan with cooking oil.

6. Arrange the gnocchi pieces in the air fryer pan. Lock the lid of the air fryer and cook for 10 minutes.

7. To serve, pour the tomato sauce over the gnocchi.

Nutritional Values per Serving:

Calories: **355** | Fat: **27.6**g | Protein: **22.1**g | Total Carbohydrates: **6.5**g | Dietary Fiber: **2.1**g | Net Carbohydrates: **4.4**g

19-Cauliflower Chao Fan Fried with Pork Pastiche

Diet Specs: GF | NF | DF

Yield: 4-servings

Serving Portion: 1 serving bowl

Preparation Time: 20 minutes

Cooking Time: 15 minutes

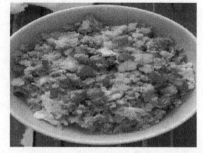

Ingredients:

½-head medium-sized cauliflower, chopped into small cubes

2-pcs eggs

2-cloves garlic, chopped

2-cups pork belly, cut into thin strips

3-pcs green capsicums

2-bulbs onions

1-tbsp soy sauce, gluten-free

1-tsp black sesame seeds

1-tbsp spring onion, chopped

1-tsp pickled ginger

Directions:

1. Place the chopped cauliflower in your food processor; pulse into smaller granules. Set aside.

2. Whisk the eggs, and swirl in the frying pan. Cook for 3 minutes.

3. Add the pork belly strips and the cauliflower rice. Stir in the onions and soy sauce. Cook for about 10 minutes.

4. To serve, distribute the preparation equally between four serving bowls. Garnish with sesame seeds, spring onions, and pickled ginger.

Nutritional Values per Serving:

Calories: **460** | Fat: **35.7**g | Protein: **28.6**g | Total Carbohydrates: **8.3**g | Dietary Fiber: **2.3**g | Net Carbohydrates: **6**g

20-All-Avocado Stuffed with Spicy Beef Bits

Diet Specs: GF | NF

Yield: 6-servings

Serving Portion: 1-halved avocado

Preparation Time: 20 minutes

Cooking Time: 20 minutes

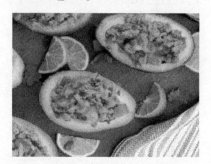

Ingredients:

1-lb. ground beef

1-tbsp chili powder

½-tsp salt

¾-tsp cumin

½-tsp dried oregano

¼-tsp garlic powder

¼-tsp onion powder

4-oz. tomato sauce, gluten-free

3-pcs medium-sized avocados, halved and pitted

1-cup cheddar cheese, shredded for garnish

¼-cup cherry tomatoes, sliced for garnish

¼-cup lettuce, shredded for garnish

A dash of chopped cilantro for garnish

Directions:

1. Cook the beef with oil and a little water in a pan for 10 minutes, stirring frequently until it turns brown. Stir in the spices and tomato sauce. Cook for another 10 minutes.

2. Load the cooked beef to each halved avocado and top with garnish.

Nutritional Values per Serving:

Calories: **280** | Fat: **23.1**g | Protein: **14**g | Total Carbohydrates: **6.3**g | Dietary Fiber: **2.2**g | Net Carbohydrates: **4.1**g

Chapter 8-Satisfying Snacks

1-Coconut Candy

Diet Specs: GF | VEG | NF | DF

Yield: 4-candy balls/1-serving

Serving Portion: 4-candy balls

Preparation Time: 10 minutes

Cooking Time: 0 minutes

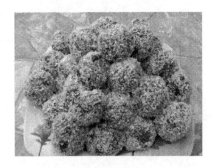

Ingredients:

2-tbsp coconut butter (or notably known as Coconut Manna)

Directions:

1. Melt the coconut butter at room temperature until it resembles a creamy butter consistency.

2. Spoon out the melted butter into candy molds. Refrigerate for 10 minutes to harden before serving.

TIP: You can make more candies and refrigerate it for several weeks placed in a closed container.

Nutritional Values per Serving:

Calories: **204** | Fat: **17.2**g | Protein: **10.2**g | Total Carbohydrates: **3**g | Dietary Fiber: **0.8**g | Net Carbohydrates: **2.2**g

2-Mozzarella Mound Munchies

Diet Specs: VEG | NF

Yield: 3-servings

Serving Portion: 1-mozzarella cheese mound

Preparation Time: 5 minutes

Cooking Time: 6 minutes

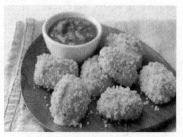

Ingredients:

⅓-cup panko bread, herb-flavored

2-pcs egg whites

6-tbsp mozzarella cheese, molded into 2-tbsp balls

¼-cup marinara sauce

Directions:

1. Preheat your oven to 425°F.

2. Toast the panko breadcrumbs for 2 minutes, stirring frequently, in a medium skillet placed over medium heat.

3. Transfer the breadcrumbs in a bowl. Add the egg whites into a separate bowl.

4. Dip a cheeseball into the egg and roll in the panko. Place the breaded cheese on a greased baking sheet, and bake for 3 minutes. Repeat the process for the remaining cheese.

5. Heat the marinara sauce in your microwave oven for half a minute. Serve the breaded cheeseball with the sauce

Nutritional Values per Serving:

Calories: **157** | Fat: **13.2**g | Protein: **5.9**g | Total Carbohydrates: **4.8**g | Dietary Fiber: **1.1**g | Net Carbohydrates: **3.7**g

3-Philadelphia Potato Praline

Diet Specs: GF | VEG | NF

Yield: 8 x 45-calorie pralines /2-servings

Serving Portion: 4-pralines

Preparation Time: 30 minutes

Cooking Time: 0 minutes

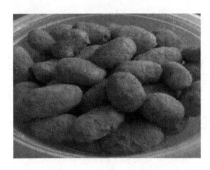

Ingredients:

⅓-cup Philadelphia cream cheese

1½-cup coconut, unsweetened and shredded

1-tbsp butter

¼-tsp ground cinnamon

Sweetener of choice

Directions:

1. Combine all the ingredients except for the ground cinnamon in a bowl. Refrigerate the mixture and allow setting until it hardens.

2. Divide the mixture into 8 portions and roll each portion into potato shapes. Place them on a sheet of parchment paper.

3. Sprinkle all over with the cinnamon and store in the fridge for a week before serving.

TIP: When making more servings, apportion the batter by its weight by summing up the total weight of the ingredients less the cinnamon, and dividing by the number of servings desired.

Nutritional Values per Serving:

Calories: **180** | Fat: **15.3**g | Protein: **8.9**g | Total Carbohydrates: **3.2**g | Dietary Fiber: **1.5**g | Net Carbohydrates: **1.7**g

4-Tasty Turkey Cheese Cylinders

Diet Specs: GF | NF

Yield: one serving

Serving Portion: 2-rollups

Preparation Time: 5 minutes

Cooking Time: 0 minutes

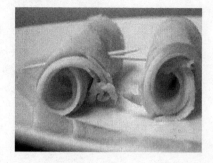

Ingredients:

1-oz. turkey, roasted and sliced

1-oz. cheese

Directions:

1. Slice the cheese into a long strip, enough to fit the turkey slice.

2. Wrap the turkey slice around the cheese.

Nutritional Values per Serving:

Calories: **162** | Fat: **10.9**g | Protein: **15.6**g | Total Carbohydrates: **3.8**g | Dietary Fiber: **0**g | Net Carbohydrates: **3.8**g

5-Fried Flaxseed Tortilla Treat

Diet Specs: VEG | NF | DF

Yield: 3-servings

Serving Portion: 2-shells flaxseed tortillas

Preparation Time: 5 minutes

Cooking Time: 10 minutes

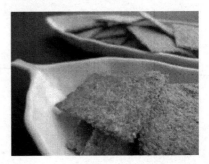

Ingredients:

6-shells flaxseed tortillas, sliced into chip-sized cuts

3-tbsp olive oil

A dash of salt and pepper

Directions:

1. Fry the flaxseed chips with olive oil in a large pan placed over medium-high heat. Cook for 10 minutes until the chips become crispy, stirring frequently. Strain the chips and place on a paper towel to drain excess oil.

2. Season the chips with a dash of salt and pepper.

Nutritional Values per Serving:

Calories: **36** | Fat: **2.8**g | Protein: **0.8**g | Total Carbohydrates: **2.7**g | Dietary Fiber: **0.7**g | Net Carbohydrates: **2**g

6-Power-Packed Butter Balls

Diet Specs: GF | VEG | DF

Yield: 10-balls/5-servings

Serving Portion: 2-butter balls

Preparation Time: 80 minutes

Cooking Time: 0 minutes

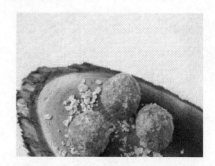

Ingredients:

2-tbsp cocoa powder + 1-tbsp for dusting

2-tbsp plain oatmeal, gluten-free

⅔-cup peanut butter or chia butter

1-tbsp organic chia seeds

3-tbsp protein powder

Directions:

1. Mix the cocoa powder, oatmeal, peanut butter chia seeds, and protein powder.

2. By using your hand, form balls from the mixture. Dust each ball with cocoa powder.

3. Place the balls in the fridge for 1 hour before serving.

Nutritional Values per Serving:

Calories: **128** | Fat: **10.1**g | Protein: **4.9**g | Total Carbohydrates: **7.2**g | Dietary Fiber: **2.9**g | Net Carbohydrates: **4.3**g

7-Choco Coco Cups

Diet Specs: GF | VEG | NF | DF

Yield: 20-mini cups/10-servings

Serving Portion: 2-mini cups

Preparation Time: 50 minutes

Cooking Time: 0 minutes

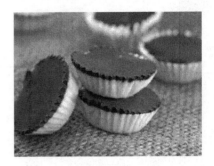

Ingredients:

For the Coconut Base:

½-cup coconut butter

½-cup coconut oil

½-cup unsweetened coconut, shredded

3-tbsp powdered sweetener

For the Chocolate Topping:

3-oz. sugar-free dark chocolate

Directions:

1. Line a muffin pan with 20 mini parchment cups.

2. Heat the coconut butter with the coconut oil in a saucepan placed over low heat. Stir until the butter melts. Stir in the shredded coconut and sweetener until fully combined.

3. Divide the mixture equally between the prepared muffin cups. Freeze for 30 minutes until firm.

4. Melt the dark chocolate and spoon over the cold filling. Let it set for 15 minutes before serving.

TIP: You can store the candy cups in your countertop for up to a week.

Nutritional Values per Serving:

Calories: **240** | Fat: **25.3**g | Protein: **2.1**g | Total Carbohydrates: **5**g | Dietary Fiber: **4**g | Net Carbohydrates: **1**g

8-Corndog Clumps

Diet Specs: GF

Yield: 20-corndogs/10-servings

Serving Portion: 2-corndogs

Preparation Time: 5 minutes

Cooking Time: 15 minutes

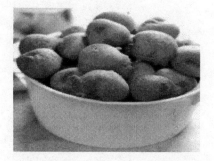

Ingredients:

¼-tsp. baking powder

¼-tsp. salt

½-cup almond flour

½-cup flaxseed meal

1-tbsp psyllium husk powder

3-packets sweetener

1-pc large egg

⅓-cup sour cream

¼-cup melted butter

¼-cup coconut milk

10-pcs (2-oz.) smoked sausage, sliced in half

Directions:

1. Preheat your oven to 375°F. Grease a 20-cup muffin pan.

2. Combine the first six ingredients in a bowl. Add the egg, sour cream, and butter and mix well. Pour in the coconut milk, and mix again. Pour the batter in the pan.

3. Insert a sliced sausage into the center of each muffin. Place the pan in the oven.

4. Bake for 12 minutes; thereafter, broil for 3 minutes, set on high heat.

Nutritional Values per Serving:

Calories: **148** | Fat: **13.2**g | Protein: **3.9**g | Total Carbohydrates: **4**g |
Dietary Fiber: **1.6**g | Net Carbohydrates: **3.4**g

9-Kingly Kale Crispy Chips

Diet Specs: GF | V | NF | DF

Yield: one -serving

Serving Portion: 1 serving bowl

Preparation Time: 0 minutes

Cooking Time: 0 minutes

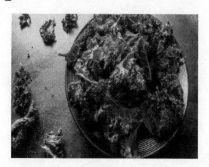

Ingredients

1-bunch large kale, rinsed, drained, and stemless

2-tbsp olive oil

1-tbsp salt

Directions:

1. Preheat your oven to 350°F.

2. Place the kale in a plastic bag. Pour the oil, and mix well by shaking the bag until coating thoroughly each leaf.

3. Spread the kale onto a baking sheet. Press the leaves flat to obtain an evenly crisped cook for each leaf.

4. Bake for 12 minutes until the edges turn brown while the rest of the kales remain dark green.

5. Sprinkle the salt over the baked kale and serve.

TIP: There is a fine line between perfect baking and overcooking the kale leaves. Overcooked kale comes out with a very bitter taste.

Nutritional Values per Serving:

Calories: **81** | Fat: **7.6**g | Protein: **1.9**g | Total Carbohydrates: **2.1**g | Dietary Fiber: **0.9**g | Net Carbohydrates: **1.2**g

10-Ambrosial Avocado Puree Pudding

Diet Specs: GF | VEG | NF | DF

Yield: 3-servings

Serving Portion: 1-glass

Preparation Time: 5 minutes

Cooking Time: 0 minutes

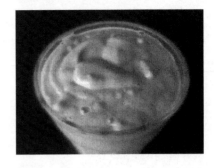

Ingredients

2-ripe Hass avocados, peeled, pitted and cut into chunks

2-tsp organic vanilla extract

80-drops of liquid sweetener

1-can (113.5-oz.) organic coconut milk

1-tbsp lime juice from organic lime

Directions

1. Combine all the ingredients in a blender. Blend to a smooth and velvety consistency. Pour the blend equally between three glasses. Chill before serving.

Nutritional Values per Serving:

Calories: **240** | Fat: **23.8**g | Protein: **2.8**g | Total Carbohydrates: **12.8**g | Dietary Fiber: **9**g | Net Carbohydrates: **3.8**g

Chapter 9-Delectable Desserts

1-Cool Cucumber Sushi with Sriracha Sauce

Diet Specs: GF | VEG | NF | DF

Yield: 12-cucumber sushi slices/4-servings

Serving Portion: 3-cucumber sushi slices

Preparation Time: 20 minutes

Cooking Time: 0 minutes

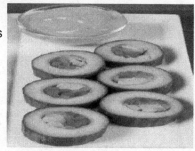

Ingredients:

For the Sushi:

2-pcs medium cucumbers

¼-pc avocado, thinly sliced

2-pcs small carrots, thinly sliced

½-pc red bell pepper, thinly sliced

½-pc yellow bell pepper, thinly sliced

For the Sriracha Sauce:

⅓-cup mayonnaise

1-tbsp sriracha

1-tsp soy sauce, gluten-free

Directions:

1. Slice one end of the cucumbers, and core them by using a small spoon to remove the seeds until completely hollow.

2. By using a butter knife, press the avocado slices into the center of each cucumber. Slide in the carrots and bell peppers until filling up completely each cucumber.

3. To make the dipping sauce, whisk to combine all the sauce ingredients in a bowl.

4. Slice the cucumber into 1"-thick round pieces, Serve with sauce on the side.

Nutritional Values per Serving:

Calories: **110** | Fat: **10.1**g | Protein: **1.9**g | Total Carbohydrates: **4.8**g | Dietary Fiber: **2**g | Net Carbohydrates: **2.8**g

2-Coco Crack Bake-less Biscuit Bars

Diet Specs: GF | V | NF | DF

Yield: 20-servings

Serving Portion: 1-bar

Preparation Time: 2 minutes

Cooking Time: 3 minutes

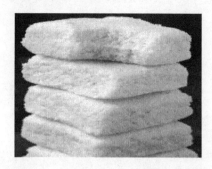

Ingredients:

3-cups unsweetened coconut flakes, shredded

1-cup coconut oil, melted

¼-cup liquid sweetener of choice

Directions:

1. Line an 8"-square baking pan with parchment paper. Set aside.

2. Combine all the ingredients in a large mixing bowl. Mix well to a thick batter. (Add a little liquid sweetener or water if the batter is too crumbly.

3. Pour and press firmly the mixture in the prepared pan. Refrigerate until firm.

4. To serve, slice the hardened mixture into 2" x 8" bars.

TIP: You can store the bars in covered jars at room temperature (covered) for up to a week; up to a month when refrigerated; and, up to a couple of months when frozen.

Nutritional Values per Serving:

Calories: **106** | Fat: **10.5**g | Protein: **2.9**g | Total Carbohydrates: **2**g | Dietary Fiber: **2**g | Net Carbohydrates: **0**g

3-Chocolate-Coated Sweet Strawberries

Diet Specs: GF | V | NF | DF

Yield: 16-candy cubes/8-servings

Serving Portion: 2-candy cubes

Preparation Time: 4 hours 10 minutes

Cooking Time: 0 minutes

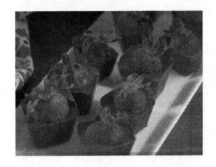

Ingredients:

2-cups melted chocolate chips, dairy-free

2-tbsp coconut oil

16-pcs fresh strawberries, with stems

Directions:

1. Combine the melted chocolate and coconut oil in a medium bowl. Mix well until fully combined.

2. Scoop the chocolate mixture into each mold of an ice cube tray. Top each with a strawberry, with its stem part up. Pour the remaining chocolate mixture over strawberries. Freeze for 4 hours until the chocolate hardens.

Nutritional Values per Serving:

Calories: **125** | Fat: **11.1**g | Protein: **2.7**g | Total Carbohydrates: **5**g | Dietary Fiber: **1.4**g | Net Carbohydrates: **3.6**g

4-Matcha Muffins with Choco-Coco Coating

Diet Specs: GF | VEG | DF

Yield: 8-muffins/4-servings

Serving Portion: 2-muffins

Preparation Time: 15 minutes

Cooking Time: 15 minutes

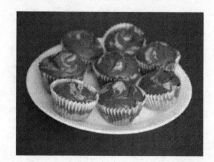

Ingredients:

½-cup almond flour

1-tbsp yeast

1-tbsp cooking matcha powder

1-tbsp cashew nuts

½-cup milk substitute with hydrogenated vegetable oil

1-tbsp peanut butter

1-tbsp cacao nibs

1-tbsp coconut syrup, gluten-free

3-tbsp milk substitute with hydrogenated vegetable oil

A handful of Goji berries (or blueberries and raspberries) and cocoa nuggets (optional)

Directions:

1. Mix the flour, yeast, matcha powder, cashews. Pour ½-cup of vegetable milk gradually while mixing into dough.

2. Put dough in a pre-greased muffin pan. Bake for 15 minutes at 350°F.

3. Mix the peanut butter with cacao, syrup, and milk to make the icing. To serve, pour the icing and garnish with cocoa nuggets and Goji berries.

Nutritional Values per Serving:

Calories: **140** | Fat: **10.9**g | Protein: **5.1**g | Total Carbohydrates: **8.8**g | Dietary Fiber: **3.4**g | Net Carbohydrates: **5.4**g

5-Cinnamon Cup Cake

Diet Specs: GF | V | NF | DF

Yield: one serving

Serving Portion: 1-cup cake

Preparation Time: 1 minute

Cooking Time: 0 minutes

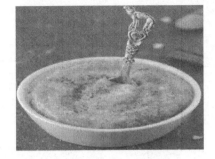

Ingredients:

1-scoop vanilla protein powder

½-tsp baking powder

1-tbsp coconut flour

½-tsp cinnamon

1-tbsp granulated sweetener of choice

¼-cup almond milk

¼-tsp vanilla extract

1-tsp granulated sweetener of choice

½-tsp cinnamon powder

For the Butter Glaze:

1-tbsp coconut butter, melted

½-tsp almond milk

A pinch of cinnamon powder

Directions:

1. Combine the protein powder, baking powder, coconut flour, cinnamon, and sweetener in a greased microwave-safe bowl. Mix well until fully combined.

2. Pour the milk, vanilla extract, and sweetener. Mix thoroughly to form a batter. (Add a little milk if the batter is too crumbly). Top with a sprinkling of cinnamon powder.

3. Cook in the microwave for 1-minute. Meanwhile, combine all the butter glaze ingredients in a bowl. To serve, top the cake with the butter glaze.

Nutritional Values per Serving:

Calories: **263** | Fat: **24.1**g | Protein: **7.6**g | Total Carbohydrates: **14.2**g | Dietary Fiber: **10.3**g | Net Carbohydrates: **3.9**g

6-Choco 'Cado Twin Truffles

Diet Specs: GF | V | NF | DF

Yield: 15-candy balls/5-servings

Serving Portion: 3-candy balls

Preparation Time: 30 minutes

Cooking Time: 0 minutes

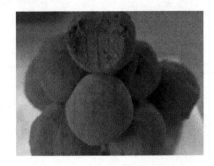

Ingredients:

1-cup melted dark chocolate chips, dairy-free

1-pc small avocado, mashed

1-tsp vanilla extract

¼-tsp kosher salt

¼-cup cocoa powder

Directions:

1. Combine the melted chocolate with avocado, vanilla, and salt in a bowl. Mix well until fully combined. Refrigerate for 20 minutes to firm up slightly.

2. By using a small spoon, scoop about a tablespoon of the chocolate mixture and roll it in the palm of your hand to form a ball. Repeat the process to consume the mixture.

3. Roll each ball in cocoa powder.

Nutritional Values per Serving:

Calories: **68** | Fat: **5.8**g | Protein: **1.6**g | Total Carbohydrates: **4.2**g | Dietary Fiber: **1.8**g | Net Carbohydrates: **2.4**g

7-Butter Ball Bombs

Diet Specs: GF | V | DF

Yield: 30-servings/10-servings

Serving Portion: 3-butter balls

Preparation Time: 65mins

Cooking Time: 0 minutes

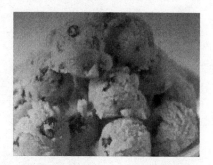

Ingredients:

8-tbsp (1 stick) butter, softened to room temperature

⅓-cup sweetener

½-tsp. pure vanilla extract

½-tsp. kosher salt

2-cups almond flour

⅔-cup unsweetened dark chocolate chips, dairy-free

Directions:

1. By using your hand mixer, beat the butter in a large bowl until light and fluffy. Add the sweetener, vanilla extract, and salt. Beat again until fully combined.

2. Add gradually the almond flour, beating continuously until no dry portions remain. Fold in the chocolate chips. Cover the bowl with a plastic wrap and refrigerate for 20 minutes to firm slightly.

3. By using a small spoon, scoop the dough to form into small balls.

TIP: You can store the balls for up to a week inside the fridge and up to a month inside the freezer.

Nutritional Values per Serving:

Calories: **51** | Fat: **4.3**g | Protein: **0.7**g | Total Carbohydrates: **2.7**g | Dietary Fiber: **0.4**g | Net Carbohydrates: **2.3**g

8-Choco Coco Cookies

Diet Specs: GF | VEG

Yield: 18-servings/6-servings

Serving Portion: 3-cookies

Preparation Time: 10 minutes

Cooking Time: 15 minutes

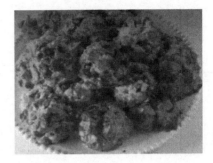

Ingredients:

¼-cup coconut oil

4-tbsp butter, softened

2-tbsp sweetener

4-pcs egg yolks

1-cup dark unsweetened chocolate chips

1-cup coconut flakes

¾-cup roughly chopped walnuts

Directions:

1. Preheat your oven to 350°F. Line a baking tray with parchment paper.

2. Combine all the ingredients in a large mixing bowl stir together coconut oil, butter, sweetener, and egg yolks. Mix in chocolate chips, coconut, and walnuts. Mix well until fully combined.

3. Form cookies out of the mixture, and place them in the baking tray. Bake for 15 minutes until golden.

Nutritional Values per Serving:

Calories: **130** | Fat: **11.5**g | Protein: **2.9**g | Total Carbohydrates: **6**g | Dietary Fiber: **2.2**g | Net Carbohydrates: **3.8**g

9-Carrot Compact Cake

Diet Specs: GF | VEG

Yield: 16-cake balls/8-servings

Serving Portion: 2-cake balls

Preparation Time: 20 minutes

Cooking Time: 0 minutes

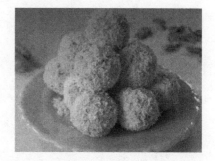

Ingredients:

1-block (8-oz.) cream cheese, softened

¾-cup coconut flour

1-tsp sweetener

½-tsp pure vanilla extract

1-tsp cinnamon

¼-tsp ground nutmeg

½-cup pecans, chopped

1-cup carrots, grated

1-cup unsweetened coconut, shredded

Directions:

1. Combine the first six ingredients in a large mixing bowl. Mix well by using a hand mixer until fully combined. Fold in the pecans and carrots.

2. Form 16 balls from the mixture, and roll each ball in shredded coconut.

Nutritional Values per Serving:

Calories: **94** | Fat: **8.3**g | Protein: **2.8**g | Total Carbohydrates: **5.2**g | Dietary Fiber: **3.1**g | Net Carbohydrates: **2.1**g

10-Chilled Cream

Diet Specs: GF | VEG | NF

Yield: 16-scoops/8-servings

Serving Portion: 2-ice cream scoops

Preparation Time: 8 hours 15 minutes

Cooking Time: 0 minutes

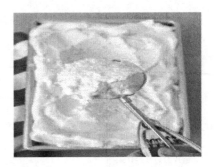

Ingredients:

2-cans (15-oz.) coconut milk, refrigerated for at least 3 hours

2-cups heavy cream

1-tsp pure vanilla extract

¼-cup sweetener

A pinch of kosher salt

Directions:

1. Spoon the refrigerated coconut milk into a large bowl. Leave the liquid in the can. By using a hand mixer, beat the milk until turning creamy. Set aside.

2. Beat the heavy cream in a separate large bowl until it forms soft peaks. Add the vanilla and sweetener. Beat again until fully combined.

3. Fold in the whipped milk into the whipped cream. Mix well and transfer the mixture in a loaf pan.

4. Place the pan in the freezer for 5 hours until the mixture becomes solid.

Nutritional Values per Serving:

Calories: **340** | Fat: **34.8**g | Protein: **3.7**g | Total Carbohydrates: **5.2**g | Dietary Fiber: **2.1**g | Net Carbohydrates: **3.1**g

Cooking Calibrations & Conversion Charts

For their popularity, all these ketogenic food recipes have found their way in a globally huge scale. This implies that they include several international versions with varying cooking measurements.

However, to facilitate your food shopping and cooking experiences, this book streamlines the cooking measurements of the recipes into the U.S. Customary Measurement Units. For further reference and convenience, the following charts present the most commonly used cooking measurements with their equivalents:

For measuring dry ingredients, measure them in graduated spoons and cups.

COMMON US DRY VOLUME MEASUREMENTS	
MEASURE	EQUIVALENT
a pinch	⅛-teaspoon
a dash	¼-teaspoon
3-teaspoons	1-Tablespoon
⅛-cup	2-Tablespoons
¼-cup	4-Tablespoons
⅓-cup	5-Tablespoons plus 1-teaspoon
½-cup	8-Tablespoons
¾-cup	12-Tablespoons
1-cup	16-Tablespoons
1-pound	16-ounces

Except with those most critical cooking procedures and preparations, the British or Imperial measurements have the slightest variations with the International or Metric System compared to U.S. units. Thus, both the Metric and Imperial Systems are relatively the same.

For measuring liquid ingredients, the customary U.S. fluid ounce and British pint differ notably. To distinguish each, take note of their conversion factors:

() Convert U.S. pints into British pints by multiplying **0.83.**

() Convert U.S. fluid ounces into British fluid ounces by multiplying **1.04.**

COMMON US LIQUID VOLUME MEASUREMENTS	
MEASURE	**EQUIVALENT**
1-ounce	28-grams
8-fluid ounces	1-cup
1-pint	2-cups
1-quart	2-pints
1-gallon	4-quarts
1-teaspoon	5-ml
1-tablespoon	15-ml
1-cup	240-ml

Additionally, here are cooking temperature charts that explain at which oven or gas temperature range is ideal for your cooking applications:

OVEN TEMPERATURE RANGE, °F	COOKING APPLICATIONS
325 – 350 normal heat range	slow cooking/braising/cake baking to ensure a Maillard reaction or the browning of proteins, as well as caramelization or the browning of sugars
375 – 400 medium-high heat	shorter term roasting/baking to ensure desirable appearances of bubbling golden cheese, crisp edges to cookies, and crisp golden skin to chicken
425 – 450 high heat	short-term roasting/baking to ensure pastries with a golden color puff
475 – 500 ultra-high heat	baking breads/pizza shells since it allows the dough to rise before the gluten has any chances to set

OVEN TEMPERATURE CONVERSION CHART		
Fahrenheit, °F	**Celsius, °C**	**Gas Mark Rating**
275	140	1-cool
300	150	2
325	165	3-very moderate
350	180	4-moderate
375	190	5
400	200	6-moderately hot
425	220	7- hot
450	230	9
475	240	10- very hot

To guide further you with other important cooking measurement conversions, check your preferences with this summarized chart:

US TO METRIC CONVERSIONS	
1/5-teaspoon	1-mL
1-teaspoon	5-ml
1-tablespoon	15-ml
1-fluid ounce	30-ml
3.4-fluid ounce	100-ml
34-fluid ounce	1-liter
1/5-cup	50-ml
1-cup	240-ml
2-cups (1-pint)	470-ml
2.1-pints	1-liter
4-cups (1-quart)	0.95-liter
4.2-cups	1-liter
1.06-quarts	1-liter
4-quarts (1-gallon)	3.8-liters
0.26-gallon	1-liter
0.035-ounce	1-gram
1-oz.	28-grams
3.5-oz.	100-grams
35-oz.	1-kilogram
1-pound	454-grams
1.10-pounds	500-grams
2.205-pounds	1-kilogram

Chapter 10-Daily Dietary Planning Programs

Plan and organize your diet; diet on your organized plan! Start to plan for seven days' worth of your ketogenic diet recipes, and you will save much of your precious time, effort, and money in the process.

Bear in mind, it would be a whole lot easier going to a restaurant or cooking an instant convenience food when everybody at home is hungry or you still have to prepare or defrost food stocks; nonetheless, a little planning will let you go a long, long way to avoid such diversions from your diet!

Your 7-day meal plan will be guiding you to program the entire duration of your scheduled daily meals while making your food shopping and cooking experiences easier than ever. All the recipes that compose your meal plan will be the recipes presented in this book.

Hence, squeeze your creative juices and explore mixing and matching up your daily cooking routines with your recipes. You should be able to look and shop for all the ingredients of the recipes since they are easily available and accessible in most supermarkets, wherever your location is. In the end, your ketogenic diet meal-planning program will be your essential tool for maintaining and sustaining your dietary change in accordance with your intended calorie consumption!

Calorie Consumption Calculation

For fitness buffs, especially when you are focusing more about total wellness with your ketogenic dietary journey, you should be aware of your *recommended daily calorie intake* (RDCI) value. You can actually calculate manually your estimated RDCI value.

You should first understand your *Basal Metabolic Rate* (BMR). The BMR is essentially the number of calories you would have been burning if you were in bed all day or not in any way performing a moderate or strenuous physical activity. However, this rate differs in gender. Initially, you calculate for your BMR by using the following formula:

INDIVIDUAL	BASAL METABOLIC RATE (BMR) FORMULA
MEN	66 + (13.7 x WEIGHT IN KILOGRAMS) + (5 x HEIGHT IN CM) – (6.8 x AGE IN YEARS)
WOMEN	65 + (9.6 x WEIGHT IN KILOGRAMS) + (1.8 x HEIGHT IN CM) – (4.7 x AGE IN YEARS)

Subsequently, you calculate for the proximate value of your RDCI by using the *Harris-Benedict Formula* (as demonstrated on the following chart). The formula actually factors the various intensity levels of your day-to-day physical activities such as your daily physical fitness training, work, and routines with respect to your calculated BMR:

DAILY ACTIVITY INTENSITY LEVEL	HARRIS-BENEDICT FORMULA
Least Active little or no exercise	BMR x 1.2
Lightly Active light exercise/work 1-3 days per week	BMR x 1.375
Moderately Active moderate exercise/work 3-5 days per week	BMR x 1.55
Very Active hard exercise/work 6-7 days a week	BMR x 1.725
Extra Active very hard exercise/work 6-7 days a week	BMR x 1.9

The following daily meal plans derive RDCI values of [1,500], [1,750], and [2,000], which will be dependent on your corresponding BMR results to help you to either maintain or reduce your weight. Your RDCI indicates how much macronutrients contained in a serving portion of food that will contribute to your daily ketogenic diet.

7-Day Dietary Planning Program (1,500 Calorie Consumption)

Starting and sticking to a daily 1,500-calorie meal plan can be challenging; however, if you only know your daily allowances for each food group or macronutrient consumption, then it can help you to know what to eat and plan a dietary program that is both nutritious and fulfilling.

To be more precise on reducing calorie intakes to help you shed off healthy pounds per week, calculate your daily calorie goal by multiplying your present weight by 12. The result denotes your basic daily calorie consumption. If your goal is to:

♥ Lose 1 pound per week, cut down 500 calories a day

♥ Lose 2 pounds per week, cut down 1,000 calories a day

Hence, if you are currently weighing 150 pounds and you aim is to lose one pound weekly, then:

150 [pounds] x 12 = 1,800 [calories]

1,800 [calories] − 500 [calories] = 1,300 calories

However, this formula assumes that you are sedentary. Otherwise, you need to take more calories than you initially calculated to feel full during the day. Your ideal gauge for whether you are indeed losing weight or at the proper level of cutting down your calories will be how satisfied you feel. You should never be hungry all day!

If you are still unsure, begin safely with a 1,500-calorie ketogenic diet plan. For, after all, this level is where most people are able to lose weight. You can eat delicious foods, albeit, low in calories while feeling full when following this easy diet meal plan:

DAY-1	KETOGENIC MEALS	SERVING PORTION	NUTRITIONAL VALUES PER SERVING	
BREAKFAST	Spinach Sausage Feta Frittata	1-frittata wedge	Calories: **295** | Fat: **22.9g** | Protein: **18.5g** | Total Carbs: **4.6g** | Dietary Fiber: **1g** | Net Carbs: **3.6g**	
SNACK	Choco Coco Cups	2-mini cups	Calories: **240** | Fat: **25.3g** | Protein: **2.1g** | Total Carbs: **5g** | Dietary Fiber: **4g** | Net Carbs: **1g**	
LUNCH	Smoky Sage Sausage	1-patty	Calories: **170** | Fat: **13.2g** | Protein: **8.4g** | Total Carbs: **5.3g** | Dietary Fiber: **1g** | Net Carbs: **4.3g**	
	Coco Crack Bake-less Biscuit Bars	1-biscuit bar	Calories: **106** | Fat: **10.5g** | Protein: **3g** | Total Carbs: **2.3g** | Dietary Fiber: **2g** | Net Carbs: **0.3g**	
SNACK	Ambrosial Avocado Puree Pudding	1-glass	Calories: **240** | Fat: **23.8g** | Protein: **2.8g** | Total Carbs: **12.8g** | Dietary Fiber: **9g** | Net Carbs: **3.8g**	
DINNER	Grain-less Gnocchi in Melted Mozzarella	1-serving bowl	Calories: **355** | Fat: **27.6g** | Protein: **22.1g** | Total Carbs: **6.5g** | Dietary Fiber: **2.1g** | Net Carbs: **4.4g**	
	Carrot Compact Cake	2-cake balls	Calories: **94** | Fat: **8.3g** | Protein: **2.8g** | Total Carbs: **5.2g** | Dietary Fiber: **3.1g** | Net Carbs: **2.1g**	
TOTAL CALORIE CONSUMPTION			1,500	
FAT			131.6g	78.9%
PROTEIN			59.7g	15.9%
NET CARBOHYDRATES			19.5g	5.2%

DAY-2	KETOGENIC MEALS	SERVING PORTION	NUTRITIONAL VALUES PER SERVING
BREAKFAST	Hearty Hodgepodge	1-serving bowl	Calories: 290 | Fat: 24g | Protein: 14.6 g | Total Carbs: 6.7g | Dietary Fiber: 3.1g | Net Carbs: 3.6g
SNACK	Coconut Candy	4-candy balls	Calories: 204 | Fat: 17.2g | Protein: 10.2g | Total Carbs: 3g | Dietary Fiber: 0.8g | Net Carbs: 2.2g
LUNCH	Pulled Pepper-Lemon Loins	1-chicken loin	Calories: 280 | Fat: 23.3g | Protein: 14g | Total Carbs: 4.1g | Dietary Fiber: 0.6g | Net Carbs: 3.5g
LUNCH	Butter Ball Bombs	3-butter balls	Calories: 51 | Fat: 4.3g | Protein: 0.7g | Total Carbs: 2.7g | Dietary Fiber: 0.4g | Net Carbs: 2.3g
SNACK	Philadelphia Potato Praline	4-pralines	Calories: 180 | Fat: 15.3g | Protein: 8.9g | Total Carbs: 3.2g | Dietary Fiber: 1.5g | Net Carbs: 1.7g
DINNER	Soba & Spinach Sprouts	1-serving bowl	Calories: 355 | Fat: 29.6g | Protein: 17.8g | Total Carbs: 8.3g | Dietary Fiber: 3.9g | Net Carbs: 4.4g
DINNER	Matcha Muffins with Choco-Coco Coating	2-muffins	Calories: 140 | Fat: 10.9g | Protein: 5.1g | Total Carbs: 8.8g | Dietary Fiber: 3.4g | Net Carbs: 5.4g
TOTAL CALORIE CONSUMPTION			1,500
FAT			124.6g — 74.8%
PROTEIN			71.3g — 19.0%
NET CARBOHYDRATES			23.1g — 6.2%

DAY-3	KETOGENIC MEALS	SERVING PORTION	NUTRITIONAL VALUES PER SERVING
BREAKFAST	Avocado Aliment with Egg Element	1-halved stuffed avocado	Calories: 275 | Fat: 23.8g | Protein: 11.8g | Total Carbs: 7.4g | Dietary Fiber: 4g | Net Carbs: 3.4g
SNACK	Power-Packed Butter Balls	2-balls	Calories: 128 | Fat: 10.1g | Protein: 4.9g | Total Carbs: 7.2g | Dietary Fiber: 2.9g | Net Carbs: 4.3g
LUNCH	Aubergine Á la Lasagna Lunch	1-lasagna slice	Calories: 346 | Fat: 27g | Protein: 21.4g | Total Carbs: 7.9g | Dietary Fiber: 3.5g | Net Carbs: 4.4g
	Chocolate-Coated Sweet Strawberries	2-candy cubes	Calories: 125 | Fat: 11.1g | Protein: 2.7g | Total Carbs: 5g | Dietary Fiber: 1.4g | Net Carbs: 3.6g
SNACK	Corndog Clumps	2-corndogs	Calories: 148 | Fat: 13.2g | Protein: 3.9g | Total Carbs: 4g | Dietary Fiber: 1.6g | Net Carbs: 3.4g
DINNER	Cheesy Cauliflower Mac Munchies	1-serving bowl	Calories: 352 | Fat: 27.8g | Protein: 20.9g | Total Carbs: 8.9g | Dietary Fiber: 4.3g | Net Carbs: 4.6g
	Choco Coco Cookies	3-cookies	Calories: 130 | Fat: 11.5g | Protein: 2.9g | Total Carbs: 6g | Dietary Fiber: 2.2g | Net Carbos: 3.8g
TOTAL CALORIE CONSUMPTION			1,504
FAT			124.5g — 74.5%
PROTEIN			68.5g — 18.2%
NET CARBOHYDRATES			27.5g — 7.3%

DAY-4	KETOGENIC MEALS	SERVING PORTION	NUTRITIONAL VALUES PER SERVING
BREAKFAST	Avocados atop Toasted Tartiné	1-tartiné	Calories: 268 | Fat: 22.4g | Protein: 13.5g | Total Carbs: 8.9g | Dietary Fiber: 6.7g | Net Carbs: 3.2g
SNACK	Tasty Turkey Cheese Cylinders	2-rollups	Calories: 162 | Fat: 10.9g | Protein: 15.6g | Total Carbs: 3.8g | Dietary Fiber: 0g | Net Carbs: 3.8g
LUNCH	Sautéed Sirloin Steak in Sour Sauce	1-serving bowl	Calories: 350 | Fat: 29.3g | Protein: 17.7g | Total Carbs: 4.9g | Dietary Fiber: 1g | Net Carbs: 3.9g
	Carrot Compact Cake	2-cake balls	Calories: 94 | Fat: 8.3g | Protein: 2.8g | Total Carbs: 5.2g | Dietary Fiber: 3.1g | Net Carbs: 2.1g
SNACK	Fried Flaxseed Tortilla Treat	2-shells flaxseed tortillas	Calories: 36 | Fat: 2.8g | Protein: 0.8g | Total Carbs: 2.7g | Dietary Fiber: 0.7g | Net Carbs: 2g
DINNER	Chicken Cauliflower Curry	1-serving bowl	Calories: 334 | Fat: 27g | Protein: 18.7g | Total Carbs: 8.4g | Dietary Fiber: 4.3g | Net Carbs: 4.1g
	Cinnamon Cup Cake	1-cup cake	Calories: 263 | Fat: 24.1g | Protein: 7.6g | Total Carbs: 14.2g | Dietary Fiber: 10.3g | Net Carbs: 3.9g
TOTAL CALORIE CONSUMPTION			1,507
FAT			124.8g — 74.5%
PROTEIN			76.7g — 20.4%
NET CARBOHYDRATES			23.0g — 6.1%

DAY-5	KETOGENIC MEALS	SERVING PORTION	NUTRITIONAL VALUES PER SERVING
BREAKFAST	Seasoned Sardines with Sunny Side	1-serving bowl	Calories: 255 | Fat: 21g | Protein: 13.5g | Total Carbs: 4.9g | Dietary Fiber: 1.8g | Net Carbs: 3.1g
SNACK	Mozzarella Mound Munchies	1-cheese mound	Calories: 157 | Fat: 13.2g | Protein: 5.9g | Total Carbs: 4.8g | Dietary Fiber: 1.1g | Net Carbs: 3.7g
LUNCH	Beef Broccoli with Sesame Sauce	1-serving bowl	Calories: 375 | Fat: 31g | Protein: 19.5g | Total Carbs: 5.4g | Dietary Fiber: 0.8g | Net Carbs: 4.6g
LUNCH	Cinnamon Cup Cake	1-cup cake	Calories: 263 | Fat: 24.1g | Protein: 7.6g | Total Carbs: 14.2g | Dietary Fiber: 10.3g | Net Carbs: 3.9g
SNACK	Kingly Kale Crispy Chips	1-serving bowl	Calories: 81 | Fat: 7.6g | Protein: 1.9g | Total Carbs: 2.1g | Dietary Fiber: 0.9g | Net Carbs: 1.2g
DINNER	Zesty Zucchini Pseudo Pasta & Sweet Spanish Onions Overload	1-serving bowl	Calories: 319 | Fat: 25.9g | Protein: 18.1g | Total Carbs: 6.6g | Dietary Fiber: 3.2g | Net Carbs: 3.4g
DINNER	Butter Ball Bombs	3-butter balls	Calories: 51 | Fat: 4.3g | Protein: 0.7g | Total Carbs: 2.7g | Dietary Fiber: 0.4g | Net Carbs: 2.3g
TOTAL CALORIE CONSUMPTION			1,501
FAT			127.1g — 76.2%
PROTEIN			67.2g — 17.9%
NET CARBOHYDRATES			22.2g — 5.9%

DAY-6	KETOGENIC MEALS	SERVING PORTION	NUTRITIONAL VALUES PER SERVING
BREAKFAST	Blueberries Breakfast Bowl	1-serving bowl	Calories: 202 | Fat: 16.8g | Protein: 10.2g | Total Carbs: 9.8g | Dietary Fiber: 5.8g | Net Carbs: 2.6g
SNACK	Ambrosial Avocado Puree Pudding	1-glass	Calories: 240 | Fat: 23.8g | Protein: 2.8g | Total Carbs: 12.8g | Dietary Fiber: 9g | Net Carbs: 3.8g
LUNCH	Chicken Curry Masala Mix	1-serving bowl	Calories: 377 | Fat: 29.3g | Protein: 23.4g | Total Carbs: 6.8g | Dietary Fiber: 1.9g | Net Carbos: 4.9g
LUNCH	Butter Ball Bombs	3-butter balls	Calories: 51 | Fat: 4.3g | Protein: 0.7g | Total Carbs: 2.7g | Dietary Fiber: 0.4g | Net Carbs: 2.3g
SNACK	Choco Coco Cups	2-mini cups	Calories: 240 | Fat: 25.3g | Protein: 2.1g | Total Carbs: 5g | Dietary Fiber: 4g | Net Carbs: 1g
DINNER	All-Avocado Stuffed with Spicy Beef Bits	1-halved stuffed avocado	Calories: 280 | Fat: 23.1g | Protein: 14g | Total Carbs: 6.3g | Dietary Fiber: 2.2g | Net Carbs: 4.1g
DINNER	Cool Cucumber Sushi with Sriracha Sauce	3-sushi slices	Calories: 110 | Fat: 10.1g | Protein: 1.9g | Total Carbs: 4.8g | Dietary Fiber: 2g | Net Carbs: 2.8g
TOTAL CALORIE CONSUMPTION		1,500	
FAT		132.7g	79.6%
PROTEIN		55.1g	14.7%
NET CARBOHYDRATES		21.5g	5.7%

DAY-7	KETOGENIC MEALS	SERVING PORTION	NUTRITIONAL VALUES PER SERVING	
BREAKFAST	Pumpkin Pancakes	2-pancakes	Calories: 200 | Fat: 16.4g | Protein: 11g | Total Carbs: 5.2g | Dietary Fiber: 3g | Net Carbs: 2.2g	
SNACK	Fried Flaxseed Tortilla Treat	2-shells flaxseed tortillas	Calories: 36 | Fat: 2.8g | Protein: 0.8g | Total Carbs: 2.7g | Dietary Fiber: 0.7g | Net Carbs: 2g	
LUNCH	Chickpeas Carrots Curry	1-serving bowl	Calories: 380 | Fat: 30.9g | Protein: 18g | Total Carbs: 14.4g | Dietary Fiber: 10.7g | Net Carbs: 3.7g	
	Matcha Muffins with Choco-Coco Coating	2-muffins	Calories: 140 | Fat: 10.9g | Protein: 5.1g | Total Carbs: 8.8g | Dietary Fiber: 3.4g | Net Carbs: 5.4g	
SNACK	Tasty Turkey Cheese Cylinders	2-rollups	Calories: 162 | Fat: 10.9g | Protein: 15.6g | Total Carbs: 3.8g | Dietary Fiber: 0g | Net Carbs: 3.8g	
DINNER	Spicy & Smoky Spinach-Set Fish Fillets	1-fish fillet	Calories: 248 | Fat: 18.8g | Protein: 15.3g | Total Carbs: 13.2g | Dietary Fiber: 8.9g | Net Carbs: 4.3g	
	Chilled Cream	2-ice cream scoops	Calories: 340 | Fat: 34.8g | Protein: 3.7g | Total Carbs: 5.2g | Dietary Fiber: 2.1g | Net Carbs: 3.1g	
TOTAL CALORIE CONSUMPTION			1,506	
FAT			125.5g	75.0%
PROTEIN			69.5g	18.5%
NET CARBOHYDRATES			24.5g	6.5%

7-Day Dietary Planning Program (1,750 Calorie Consumption)

Calorie consumption really depends on the number of calories you expend per day with your routine activities. Again, you actually base it on your weight goals.

Hence, when you are eating 1,750 calories a day, yet, only expend 1500, you will certainly gain weight. Conversely, when you are eating 1,750 calories a day, yet, expend 1900, you will definitely lose weight. As always, define your plans and keep a balance in accordance with your intents.

DAY-1	KETOGENIC MEALS	SERVING PORTION	NUTRITIONAL VALUES PER SERVING
BREAKFAST	Cream Cheese Protein Pancake	2-pancakes	Calories: 340 | Fat: 28.6g | Protein: 16.2g | Total Carbs: 8.1g | Dietary Fiber: 3.8g | Net Carbs: 4.3g
SNACKS	Choco Coco Cups	2-mini cups	Calories: 240 | Fat: 25.3g | Protein: 2.1g | Total Carbs: 5g | Dietary Fiber: 4g | Net Carbs: 1g
LUNCH	Crispy Chicken Packed in Pandan	1-chicken thigh	Calories: 382 | Fat: 32.5g | Protein: 17.8g | Total Carbs: 7.7g | Dietary Fiber: 3.1g | Net Carbs: 4.6g
	Choco 'Cado Twin Truffles	3-candy balls	Calories: 68 | Fat: 5.8g | Protein: 1.6g | Total Carbs: 4.2g | Dietary Fiber: 1.8g | Net Carbs: 2.4g
SNACKS	Philadelphia Potato Praline	4-pralines	Calories: 180 | Fat: 15.3g | Protein: 8.9g | Total Carbs: 3.2g | Dietary Fiber: 1.5g | Net Carbs: 1.7g
DINNER	Therapeutic Turmeric & Shirataki Soup	1-serving bowl	Calories: 415 | Fat: 34.6g | Protein: 21.6g | Total Carbs: 10.1g | Dietary Fiber: 5.7g | Net Carbs: 4.4g
	Chocolate-Coated Sweet Strawberries	2-candy cubes	Calories: 125 | Fat: 11.1g | Protein: 2.7g | Total Carbs: 5g | Dietary Fiber: 1.4g | Net Carbs: 3.6g
TOTAL CALORIE CONSUMPTION			1,750
FAT			153.2g | 78.8%
PROTEIN			70.9g | 16.2%
NET CARBOHYDRATES			22.0g | 5.0%

DAY-2	KETOGENIC MEALS	SERVING PORTION	NUTRITIONAL VALUES PER SERVING	
BREAKFAST	Feta-Filled Tomato-Topped Oldie Omelet	1-omelet	Calories: 335 | Fat: 28.4g | Protein: 16.2g | Total Carbs: 4.5g | Dietary Fiber: 0.8g | Net Carbs: 3.7g	
SNACKS	Ambrosial Avocado Puree Pudding	1-glass	Calories: 240 | Fat: 23.8g | Protein: 2.8g | Total Carbs: 12.8g | Dietary Fiber: 9g | Net Carbs: 3.8g	
LUNCH	Tasty Tofu Carrots &Cauliflower Cereal	1-serving bowl	Calories: 390 | Fat: 32.6g | Protein: 19.5g | Total Carbs: 17.4g | Dietary Fiber: 12.7g | Net Carbs: 4.7g	
	Coco Crack Bake-less Bounty Bars	1-bar	Calories: 106 | Fat: 10.5g | Protein: 2.9g | Total Carbs: 2g | Dietary Fiber: 2g | Net Carbs: 0g	
SNACKS	Mozzarella Mound Munchies	1-cheese mound	Calories: 157 | Fat: 13.2g | Protein: 5.9g | Total Carbs: 4.8g | Dietary Fiber: 1.1g | Net Carbs: 3.7g	
DINNER	A la Spaghetti with Asian Sauce	1-serving plate	Calories: 412 | Fat: 34.4g | Protein: 20.9g | Total Carbs: 10.5g | Dietary Fiber: 5.7g | Net Carbs: 4.8g	
	Cool Cucumber Sushi with Sriracha Sauce	3-sushi slices	Calories: 110 | Fat: 10.1g | Protein: 1.9g | Total Carbs: 4.8g | Dietary Fiber: 2g | Net Carbs: 2.8g	
TOTAL CALORIE CONSUMPTION			1,750	
FAT			153.0g	78.6%
PROTEIN			70.1g	16.0%
NET CARBOHYDRATES			23.5g	5.4%

DAY-3	KETOGENIC MEALS	SERVING PORTION	NUTRITIONAL VALUES PER SERVING
BREAKFAST	Whole-Wheat Plain Pancakes	2-pancakes	Calories: **329** | Fat: **27.6g** | Protein: **16.1g** | Total Carbs: **5.4g** | Dietary Fiber: **1.3g** | Net Carbs: **4.4g**
SNACKS	Coconut Candy	4-candy balls	Calories: **204** | Fat: **17.2g** | Protein: **10.2g** | Total Carbs: **3g** | Dietary Fiber: **0.8g** | Net Carbs: **2.2g**
LUNCH	Steamed Salmon & Salad Bento Box	1-bento box	Calories: **391** | Fat: **30.4g** | Protein: **24.9g** | Total Carbs: **11.8g** | Dietary Fiber: **7.3g** | Net Carbs: **4.5g**
	Chocolate-Coated Sweet Strawberries	2-candy cubes	Calories: **125** | Fat: **11.1g** | Protein: **2.7g** | Total Carbs: **5g** | Dietary Fiber: **1.4g** | Net Carbs: **3.6g**
SNACKS	Fried Flaxseed Tortilla Treat	2-shells flaxseed tortillas	Calories: **36** | Fat: **2.8g** | Protein: **0.8g** | Total Carbs: **2.7g** | Dietary Fiber: **0.7g** | Net Carbs: **2g**
DINNER	Cheddar Chicken Casserole	1-serving plate	Calories: **405** | Fat: **33.8g** | Protein: **22.7g** | Total Carbs: **3.6g** | Dietary Fiber: **1g** | Net Carbs: **2.6g**
	Cinnamon Cup Cake	1-cup cake	Calories: **263** | Fat: **24.1g** | Protein: **7.6g** | Total Carbs: **14.2g** | Dietary Fiber: **10.3g** | Net Carbs: **3.9g**
TOTAL CALORIE CONSUMPTION			1,753
FAT			147.0g	75.4%
PROTEIN			85.0g	19.3%
NET CARBOHYDRATES			23.2g	5.3%

DAY-4	KETOGENIC MEALS	SERVING PORTION	NUTRITIONAL VALUES PER SERVING
BREAKFAST	Romantic Raspberry Power Pancake	2-pancakes	Calories: 323 | Fat: 25.3g | Protein: 15.7g | Total Carbs: 12g | Dietary Fiber: 3.8g | Net Carbs: 4.8g
SNACKS	Tasty Turkey Cheese Cylinders	2-rollups	Calories: 162 | Fat: 10.9g | Protein: 15.6g | Total Carbs: 3.8g | Dietary Fiber: 0g | Net Carbs: 3.8g
LUNCH	Prawn Pasta	1-serving plate	Calories: 393 | Fat: 32.8g | Protein: 19.7g | Total Carbs: 14.9g | Dietary Fiber: 10.1g | Net Carbs: 4.8g
	Chilled Cream	2-ice cream scoops	Calories: 340 | Fat: 34.8g | Protein: 3.7g | Total Carbs: 5.2g | Dietary Fiber: 2.1g | Net Carbs: 3.1g
SNACKS	Kingly Kale Crispy Chips	1-serving bowl	Calories: 81 | Fat: 7.6g | Protein: 1.9g | Total Carbs: 2.1g | Dietary Fiber: 0.9g | Net Carbs: 1.2g
DINNER	Sugar Snap Pea Pods with Coco Crunch	1-serving bowl	Calories: 389 | Fat: 31.3g | Protein: 22g | Total Carbs: 7.2g | Dietary Fiber: 2.3g | Net Carbs: 4.9g
	Choco 'Cado Twin Truffles	3-candy balls	Calories: 68 | Fat: 5.8g | Protein: 1.6g | Total Carbs: 4.2g | Dietary Fiber: 1.8g | Net Carbs: 2.4g
TOTAL CALORIE CONSUMPTION			1,756
FAT			148.5g | 76.1%
PROTEIN			80.2g | 18.2%
NET CARBOHYDRATES			25.0g | 5.7%

DAY-5	KETOGENIC MEALS	SERVING PORTION	NUTRITIONAL VALUES PER SERVING	
BREAKFAST	Spinach Shoots Mediterranean Medley	1-serving bowl	Calories: 308 | Fat: 26g | Protein: 15.4g | Total Carbs: 9.7g | Dietary Fiber: 6.5g | Net Carbs: 3.2g	
SNACKS	Choco Coco Cups	2-mini cups	Calories: 240 | Fat: 25.3g | Protein: 2.1g | Total Carbs: 5g | Dietary Fiber: 4g | Net Carbs: 1g	
LUNCH	Flaky Fillets with Garden Greens	1-fish fillet	Calories: 395 | Fat: 33g | Protein: 19.8g | Total Carbs: 8.7g | Dietary Fiber: 3.9g | Net Carbs: 4.8g	
	Matcha Muffins with Choco-Coco Coating	2-muffins	Calories: 140 | Fat: 10.9g | Protein: 5.1g | Total Carbs: 8.8g | Dietary Fiber: 3.4g | Net Carbs: 5.4g	
SNACKS	Mozzarella Mound Munchies	1-cheese mound	Calories: 157 | Fat: 13.2g | Protein: 5.9g | Total Carbs: 4.8g | Dietary Fiber: 1.1g | Net Carbs: 3.7g	
DINNER	Pizza Pie with Cheesy Cauliflower Crust	2-pizza wedges	Calories: 384 | Fat: 32.1g | Protein: 19.9g | Total Carbs: 5.5g | Dietary Fiber: 1.7g | Net Carbs: 3.8g	
	Choco Coco Cookies	3-cookies	Calories: 130 | Fat: 11.5g | Protein: 2.9g | Total Carbs: 6g | Dietary Fiber: 2.2g | Net Carbos: 3.8g	
TOTAL CALORIE CONSUMPTION			1,754	
FAT			152.0 g	78.0%
PROTEIN			71.1 g	16.2%
NET CARBOHYDRATES			25.7 g	5.8%

DAY-6	KETOGENIC MEALS	SERVING PORTION	NUTRITIONAL VALUES PER SERVING	
BREAKFAST	Fish Fillet & Perky Potato Cheese Combo	1-serving plate	Calories: **298** | Fat: **24.9**g | Protein: **14.2**g | Total Carbs: **6.5**g | Dietary Fiber: **3.2**g | Net Carbs: **4.3**g	
SNACKS	Kingly Kale Crispy Chips	1-serving bowl	Calories: **81** | Fat: **7.6**g | Protein: **1.9**g | Total Carbs: **2.1**g | Dietary Fiber: **0.9**g | Net Carbs: **1.2**g	
LUNCH	Milano Meatballs with Tangy Tomato	2-meatballs	Calories: **396** | Fat: **32.6**g | Protein: **20.9**g | Total Carbs: **8.2**g | Dietary Fiber: **3.4**g | Net Carbs: **4.8**g	
	Choco Coco Cookies	3-cookies	Calories: **130** | Fat: **11.5**g | Protein: **2.9**g | Total Carbs: **6**g | Dietary Fiber: **2.2**g | Net Carbos: **3.8**g	
SNACKS	Power-Packed Butter Balls	2-balls	Calories: **128** | Fat: **10.1**g | Protein: **4.9**g | Total Carbs: **7.2**g | Dietary Fiber: **2.9**g | Net Carbs: **4.3**g	
DINNER	Spaghetti-Styled Zesty Zucchini with Guacamole Garnish	1-set guacamole and carbonara	Calories: **381** | Fat: **31.8**g | Protein: **19**g | Total Carbs: **14.3**g | Dietary Fiber: **9.5**g | Net Carbs: **4.8**g	
	Chilled Cream	2-ice cream scoops	Calories: **340** | Fat: **34.8**g | Protein: **3.7**g | Total Carbs: **5.2**g | Dietary Fiber: **2.1**g | Net Carbs: **3.1**g	
TOTAL CALORIE CONSUMPTION			1,754	
FAT			153.3g	78.6%
PROTEIN			67.5g	15.4%
NET CARBOHYDRATES			26.3g	6.0%

DAY-7	KETOGENIC MEALS	SERVING PORTION	NUTRITIONAL VALUES PER SERVING	
BREAKFAST	Mayonnaise Mixed with Energy Egg	1-serving bowl	Calories: **295**	Fat: **22.7g**	Protein: **18.8g**	Total Carbs: **3.8g**	Dietary Fiber: **0.1g**	Net Carbs: **3.7g**	
SNACKS	Choco Coco Cups	2-mini cups	Calories: **240**	Fat: **25.3g**	Protein: **2.1g**	Total Carbs: **5g**	Dietary Fiber: **4g**	Net Carbs: **1g**	
LUNCH	Stuffed Straw Mushroom Mobcap	1-cup stuffed mushroom	Calories: **401**	Fat: **34.7g**	Protein: **17.2g**	Total Carbs: **16.9g**	Dietary Fiber: **11.4g**	Net Carbs: **5g**	
	Cool Cucumber Sushi with Sriracha Sauce	3-sushi slices	Calories: **110**	Fat: **10.1g**	Protein: **1.9g**	Total Carbs: **4.8g**	Dietary Fiber: **2g**	Net Carbs: **2.8g**	
SNACKS	Ambrosial Avocado Puree Pudding	1-glass	Calories: **240**	Fat: **23.8g**	Protein: **2.8g**	Total Carbs: **12.8g**	Dietary Fiber: **9g**	Net Carbs: **3.8g**	
DINNER	Spicy Shrimps & Sweet Shishito	1-serving bowl	Calories: **370**	Fat: **28.9g**	Protein: **23g**	Total Carbs: **7.2g**	Dietary Fiber: **2.8g**	Net Carbs: **4.4g**	
	Carrot Compact Cake	2-cake balls	Calories: **94**	Fat: **8.3g**	Protein: **2.8g**	Total Carbs: **5.2g**	Dietary Fiber: **3.1g**	Net Carbs: **2.1g**	
TOTAL CALORIE CONSUMPTION			1,750	
FAT			153.8g	79.1%
PROTEIN			68.6g	15.7%
NET CARBOHYDRATES			22.8g	5.2%

7- Day Dietary Planning Program (2,000 Calorie Consumption)

For all intents of providing the most helpful nutritional information to consumers, the Food and Drug Administration (FDA) of the U.S. uses a 2,000-calorie regimen as the standard model for the entire *Nutrition Facts* label on foods. The label generally provides information about *Percentage Daily Value* (%-DV).

However, the model is not a recommendation that you ought to consume 2,000 calories a day. Moreover, it does not indicate that a 2,000-calorie regimen is worse or necessarily better than, say, a 2,500-calorie or a 1,200-calorie diet. As your constant reminder, if you were trying to gain or lose weight with the facilitation of the ketogenic diet, then you would simply adjust your daily caloric intake to reach your specific health goals.

DAY-1	KETOGENIC MEALS	SERVING PORTION	NUTRITIONAL VALUES PER SERVING	
BREAKFAST	Choco Chip Whey Waffles	2-waffles	Calories: **423** | Fat: **32.8g** | Protein: **26.5g** | Total Carbs: **8.3g** | Dietary Fiber: **2.9g** | Net Carbs: **5.4g**	
SNACKS	Ambrosial Avocado Puree Pudding	1-glass	Calories: **240** | Fat: **23.8g** | Protein: **2.8g** | Total Carbs: **12.8g** | Dietary Fiber: **9g** | Net Carbs: **3.8g**	
LUNCH	Stuffed Straw Mushroom Mobcap	1-cup stuffed mushroom	Calories: **401** | Fat: **34.7g** | Protein: **17.2g** | Total Carbs: **16.9g** | Dietary Fiber: **11.4g** | Net Carbs: **5g**	
	Coco Crack Bake-less Bounty Bars	1-bar	Calories: **106** | Fat: **10.5g** | Protein: **2.9g** | Total Carbs: **2g** | Dietary Fiber: **2g** | Net Carbs: **0g**	
SNACKS	Choco Coco Cups	2-mini cups	Calories: **240** | Fat: **25.3g** | Protein: **2.1g** | Total Carbs: **5g** | Dietary Fiber: **4g** | Net Carbs: **1g**	
DINNER	Cauliflower Chao Fan Fried with Pork Pastiche	1-serving bowl	Calories: **460** | Fat: **35.7g** | Protein: **28.6g** | Total Carbs: **8.3g** | Dietary Fiber: **2.3g** | Net Carbs: **6g**	
	Choco Coco Cookies	3-cookies	Calories: **130** | Fat: **11.5g** | Protein: **2.9g** | Total Carbs: **6g** | Dietary Fiber: **2.2g** | Net Carbos: **3.8g**	
TOTAL CALORIE CONSUMPTION			2,000	
FAT			174.3g	78.4%
PROTEIN			83.0g	16.6%
NET CARBOHYDRATES			25.0g	5.0%

DAY-2	KETOGENIC MEALS	SERVING PORTION	NUTRITIONAL VALUES PER SERVING	
BREAKFAST	Magdalena Muffins with Tart Tomatoes	2-muffins	Calories: **405** | Fat: **33.3g** | Protein: **20.3g** | Total Carbs: **11g** | Dietary Fiber: **4.9g** | Net Carbs: **6.1g**	
SNACKS	Corndog Clumps	2-corndogs	Calories: **148** | Fat: **13.2g** | Protein: **3.9g** | Total Carbs: **4g** | Dietary Fiber: **1.6g** | Net Carbs: **3.4g**	
LUNCH	Stuffed Spaghetti Squash	1-halved stuffed squash	Calories: **404** | Fat: **33.2g** | Protein: **20.3g** | Total Carbs: **7g** | Dietary Fiber: **1g** | Net Carbs: **6g**	
	Matcha Muffins with Choco-Coco Coating	2-muffins	Calories: **140** | Fat: **10.9g** | Protein: **5.1g** | Total Carbs: **8.8g** | Dietary Fiber: **3.4g** | Net Carbs: **5.4g**	
SNACKS	Philadelphia Potato Praline	4-pralines	Calories: **180** | Fat: **15.3g** | Protein: **8.9g** | Total Carbs: **3.2g** | Dietary Fiber: **1.5g** | Net Carbs: **1.7g**	
DINNER	Chickpeas & Carrot Consommé	1-serving bowl	Calories: **460** | Fat: **38.2g** | Protein: **23.3g** | Total Carbs: **10.1g** | Dietary Fiber: **4.3g** | Net Carbs: **5.8g**	
	Cinnamon Cup Cake	1-cup cake	Calories: **263** | Fat: **24.1g** | Protein: **7.6g** | Total Carbs: **14.2g** | Dietary Fiber: **10.3g** | Net Carbs: **3.9g**	
TOTAL CALORIE CONSUMPTION			2,000	
FAT			168.2g	75.7%
PROTEIN			89.4g	17.8%
NET CARBOHYDRATES			32.3g	6.5%

DAY-3	KETOGENIC MEALS	SERVING PORTION	NUTRITIONAL VALUES PER SERVING
BREAKFAST	Ave Avocado Super Smoothie	1-serving bowl	Calories: 398 | Fat: 33.1g | Protein: 20g | Total Carbs: 15.5g | Dietary Fiber: 10.6g | Net Carbs: 4.9g
SNACKS	Tasty Turkey Cheese Cylinders	2-rollups	Calories: 162 | Fat: 10.9g | Protein: 15.6g | Total Carbs: 3.8g | Dietary Fiber: 0g | Net Carbs: 3.8g
LUNCH	Shrimps & Spinach Spaghetti	1-serving plate	Calories: 425 | Fat: 33g | Protein: 25g | Total Carbs: 15.7g | Dietary Fiber: 10.4g | Net Carbs: 5.3g
	Chilled Cream	2-ice cream scoops	Calories: 340 | Fat: 34.8g | Protein: 3.7g | Total Carbs: 5.2g | Dietary Fiber: 2.1g | Net Carbs: 3.1g
SNACKS	Philadelphia Potato Praline	4-pralines	Calories: 180 | Fat: 15.3g | Protein: 8.9g | Total Carbs: 3.2g | Dietary Fiber: 1.5g | Net Carbs: 1.7g
DINNER	Charred Chicken with Squash Seed Sauce	2-chicken skewers	Calories: 428 | Fat: 35.6g | Protein: 21g | Total Carbs: 16.9g | Dietary Fiber: 11.6g | Net Carbs: 5.3g
	Choco 'Cado Twin Truffles	3-candy balls	Calories: 68 | Fat: 5.8g | Protein: 1.6g | Total Carbs: 4.2g | Dietary Fiber: 1.8g | Net Carbs: 2.4g
TOTAL CALORIE CONSUMPTION			2,001	
FAT			168.5g	75.7%
PROTEIN			95.8g	19.1%
NET CARBOHYDRATES			26.5g	5.2%

DAY-4	KETOGENIC MEALS	SERVING PORTION	NUTRITIONAL VALUES PER SERVING
BREAKFAST	Coco Cinnamon-Packed Pancakes	2-pancakes	Calories: 392 | Fat: 32.5g | Protein: 20g | Total Carbs: 11.3g | Dietary Fiber: 6.4g | Net Carbs: 4.9g
SNACKS	Kingly Kale Crispy Chips	1-serving bowl	Calories: 81 | Fat: 7.6g | Protein: 1.9g | Total Carbs: 2.1g | Dietary Fiber: 0.9g | Net Carbs: 1.2g
LUNCH	Bun-less Bacon Burger	1-bacon burger	Calories: 435 | Fat: 36.3g | Protein: 21.7g | Total Carbs: 6.1g | Dietary Fiber: 0.7g | Net Carbs: 5.4g
	Chocolate-Coated Sweet Strawberries	2-candy cubes	Calories: 125 | Fat: 11.1g | Protein: 2.7g | Total Carbs: 5g | Dietary Fiber: 1.4g | Net Carbs: 3.6g
SNACKS	Coconut Candy	4-candy balls	Calories: 204 | Fat: 17.2g | Protein: 10.2g | Total Carbs: 3g | Dietary Fiber: 0.8g | Net Carbs: 2.2g
DINNER	Shirataki & Soy Sprouts Pad Thai with Peanut Tidbits	1-serving bowl	Calories: 423 | Fat: 35.2g | Protein: 21g | Total Carbs: 14.9g | Dietary Fiber: 9.6g | Net Carbs: 5.3g
	Chilled Cream	2-ice cream scoops	Calories: 340 | Fat: 34.8g | Protein: 3.7g | Total Carbs: 5.2g | Dietary Fiber: 2.1g | Net Carbs: 3.1g
TOTAL CALORIE CONSUMPTION		2,000	
FAT		174.7g	78.6%
PROTEIN		81.2g	16.3%
NET CARBOHYDRATES		25.7g	5.1%

DAY-5	KETOGENIC MEALS	SERVING PORTION	NUTRITIONAL VALUES PER SERVING
BREAKFAST	Chocolate Chia Plain Pudding	1-serving bowl	Calories: 370 | Fat: 28.7g | Protein: 22.3g | Total Carbs: 10.8g | Dietary Fiber: 5.2g | Net Carbs: 5.6g
SNACKS	Choco Coco Cups	2-mini cups	Calories: 240 | Fat: 25.3g | Protein: 2.1g | Total Carbs: 5g | Dietary Fiber: 4g | Net Carbs: 1g
LUNCH	Poultry Pâté & Creamy Crackers	3-crackers topped with pate	Calories: 437 | Fat: 36.4g | Protein: 21.9g | Total Carbs: 5.5g | Dietary Fiber: 0g | Net Carbs: 5.5g
	Choco 'Cado Twin Truffles	3-candy balls	Calories: 68 | Fat: 5.8g | Protein: 1.6g | Total Carbs: 4.2g | Dietary Fiber: 1.8g | Net Carbs: 2.4g
SNACKS	Power-Packed Butter Balls	2-balls	Calories: 128 | Fat: 10.1g | Protein: 4.9g | Total Carbs: 7.2g | Dietary Fiber: 2.9g | Net Carbs: 4.3g
DINNER	Fresh Fettuccine with Pumpkin Pesto	1-serving bowl	Calories: 417 | Fat: 34.7g | Protein: 20.9g | Total Carbs: 10.5g | Dietary Fiber: 5.3g | Net Carbs: 5.2g
	Chilled Cream	2-ice cream scoops	Calories: 340 | Fat: 34.8g | Protein: 3.7g | Total Carbs: 5.2g | Dietary Fiber: 2.1g | Net Carbs: 3.1g
TOTAL CALORIE CONSUMPTION			2,000
FAT		175.8g	79.1%
PROTEIN		77.4g	15.5%
NET CARBOHYDRATES		27.1g	5.4%

DAY-6	KETOGENIC MEALS	SERVING PORTION	NUTRITIONAL VALUES PER SERVING
BREAKFAST	Veggie Variety with Peanut Paste	1-serving bowl	Calories: 349 | Fat: 28.7g | Protein: 18.4g | Total Carbs: 10.8g | Dietary Fiber: 6.5g | Net Carbs: 4.3g
SNACKS	Ambrosial Avocado Puree Pudding	1-glass	Calories: 240 | Fat: 23.8g | Protein: 2.8g | Total Carbs: 12.8g | Dietary Fiber: 9g | Net Carbs: 3.8g
LUNCH	Single Skillet Seafood-Filled Frittata	1-frittata wedge	Calories: 459 | Fat: 38.2g | Protein: 22.9g | Total Carbs: 8.7g | Dietary Fiber: 3g | Net Carbs: 5.7g
LUNCH	Carrot Compact Cake	2-cake balls	Calories: 94 | Fat: 8.3g | Protein: 2.8g | Total Carbs: 5.2g | Dietary Fiber: 3.1g | Net Carbs: 2.1g
SNACKS	Philadelphia Potato Praline	4-pralines	Calories: 180 | Fat: 15.3g | Protein: 8.9g | Total Carbs: 3.2g | Dietary Fiber: 1.5g | Net Carbs: 1.7g
DINNER	Therapeutic Turmeric & Shirataki Soup	1-serving bowl	Calories: 415 | Fat: 34.6g | Protein: 21.6g | Total Carbs: 10.1g | Dietary Fiber: 5.7g | Net Carbs: 4.4g
DINNER	Cinnamon Cup Cake	1-cup cake	Calories: 263 | Fat: 24.1g | Protein: 7.6g | Total Carbs: 14.2g | Dietary Fiber: 10.3g | Net Carbs: 3.9g
TOTAL CALORIE CONSUMPTION			2,000
FAT			174.6g — 77.8%
PROTEIN			85.0 g — 17.0%
NET CARBOHYDRATES			25.1g — 5.2%

DAY-7	KETOGENIC MEALS	SERVING PORTION	NUTRITIONAL VALUES PER SERVING
BREAKFAST	Cream Cheese Protein Pancake	2-pancakes	Calories: 340 | Fat: 28.1g | Protein: 16.2g | Total Carbs: 8.1g | Dietary Fiber: 3.8g | Net Carbs: 4.3g
SNACKS	Power-Packed Butter Balls	2-butter balls	Calories: 128 | Fat: 10.1g | Protein: 4.9g | Total Carbs: 7.2g | Dietary Fiber: 2.9g | Net Carbs: 4.3g
LUNCH	Baked Broccoli in Olive Oil	1-serving bowl	Calories: 484 | Fat: 39.2g | Protein: 26.7g | Total Carbs: 21.6g | Dietary Fiber: 16.8g | Net Carbs: 4.8g
LUNCH	Cool Cucumber Sushi with Sriracha Sauce	3-sushi slices	Calories: 110 | Fat: 10.1g | Protein: 1.9g | Total Carbs: 4.8g | Dietary Fiber: 2g | Net Carbs: 2.8g
SNACKS	Corndog Clumps	2-corndogs	Calories: 148 | Fat: 13.2g | Protein: 3.9g | Total Carbs: 4g | Dietary Fiber: 1.6g | Net Carbs: 3.4g
DINNER	Roasted Rib-eye Skillet Steak	1-slice rib-eye steak	Calories: 722 | Fat: 60.2g | Protein: 45g | Total Carbs: 0g | Dietary Fiber: 0g | Net Carbs: 0g
DINNER	Choco 'Cado Twin Truffles	3-candy balls	Calories: 68 | Fat: 5.8g | Protein: 1.6g | Total Carbs: 4.2g | Dietary Fiber: 1.8g | Net Carbs: 2.4g
TOTAL CALORIE CONSUMPTION		2,000	
FAT		166.7g	75.0%
PROTEIN		100.2 g	20.0%
NET CARBOHYDRATES		22.0g	5.0%

Conclusion

The ketogenic diet is neither a current fad nor a passing trend. Fact is that the ketogenic diet is a lot more powerful than those fundamentals suggested by some trendy and more popular regimen. At present, medical studies and research continue to explore and discover more about nutritional ketosis in particular and the ketogenic diet in general for further benefits and applications that they may bestow to the rest of humankind.

Contrary to what most people and pseudo-experts perceive about the diet, it is also noteworthy that the ketogenic diet is not a high-protein regimen. It is essentially a high-fat diet with a substantially reduced carbohydrate allowance and moderated protein consumptions.

As a summary, the quintessential ketogenic food composition generally consists of smaller quantities of protein, greater contents of organic or natural fats, and ample amounts of dark, green, leafy vegetables. Its concept and working principle behind is to use ketones as an alternative energy source of the body.

Upon digesting foods that contain carbohydrates, your body breaks them down into glucose. With greater carbohydrate consumptions, your blood sugar level increases, indicating an overabundance of glucose. For diabetics, they clearly understand that having high blood sugar levels from eating more carbohydrates is harmful to the body.

Therefore, your intake of more fats and lesser carbohydrates with regulated protein consumptions will eventually result in switching your body's usual metabolism process. In particular, it taps and uses your stored fats to convert them into energy instead of burning glucose or sugar, or generally, carbohydrates. Such a normal metabolic shift creates more ketone bodies while at the same time, lowering blood sugar levels and insulin production in your liver.

As glucose levels drop and ketone bodies increase in number and dominate along your bloodstream, all of your major body organs like your heart, brain, muscles, and other body cells ultimately cease to burn sugar. Left with no choice, they would rather use the ketone bodies as a substitute fuel source that leads to establishing nutritional or optimal ketosis. In other words, your body virtually becomes a fat-burning machine!

Once your body applies the ketones as principal fuel sources, a myriad of beneficial effects ensue. Thus, the bottom line of the ketogenic diet is for you to reap all the rewards of the regimen by simply switching your body to ketosis through altering the way you eat.

When implementing the dietary program properly, the keto diet is capable of being a potent regulator of metabolic disorders. Both anti-oxidant and anti-inflammatory effects of nutritional ketosis alone have always proved to be potent.

Foremost, engaging with the ketone producing, low-carb, and high-fat diet helps to shed off excess weight, strengthen and tone your muscles, enhance your moods, slow down your aging process, lowers your cholesterol levels, and boosting your energy levels.

More importantly, the ketogenic diet creates a massive impact on your general health and wellbeing since it addresses a broad spectrum of health issues, as well as several symptoms associated with inflammatory diseases. Indeed, while you are constantly under the state of ketosis, not only does it augment in the treatment of several serious health problems but also, it enables you to live a more confident, hassle-free, fulfilling and happier life.

To learn how to lose weight and stay fit needs a lot of skill that you will use for a lifetime to keep your body in tip-top shape for the sake of your health and well-being. This book points you towards going to the right direction with a no-arbitrary approach to losing weight in a healthy way. It further provides you with the proper guidance of implementing the regimen via a strategic meal-planning program while using exclusively keto-diet recipes that will enable losing weight in the most natural and simplest way.

Thanks to the proper guidance from a group of certified weight loss experts that the writer collaborated with all this time. You will lose fat and stay fit for life. Have a good luck! Get started with your ketogenic diet! We know you can do it! It is time to shed off those extra pounds. As with any other meal plans, always consult your physician before taking part in a diet plan.

References

[1]USDA Dietary Reference Intakes for Energy, Carbohydrate, Fiber, Fat, Fatty Acids, Cholesterol, Protein, and Amino Acids (page 275)

[2]Hashimoto Y, Fukuda T, Oyabu C, et al. Impact of low-carbohydrate diet on body composition: a meta-analysis of randomized controlled studies. Obes Rev. 2016;17(6):499-509

[3]Bueno NB, De Melo IS, De Oliveira SL, Da Rocha Ataide T. Very-low-carbohydrate ketogenic diet v. low-fat diet for long-term weight loss: a meta-analysis of randomized controlled trials. Br J Nutr. 2013;110(7):1178-87.

[4]Brehm BJ, Seeley RJ, Daniels SR, D'alessio DA. A randomized trial comparing a very low carbohydrate diet and a calorie-restricted low-fat diet on body weight and cardiovascular risk factors in healthy women. J Clin Endocrinol Metab. 2003;88(4):1617-23.

[5]Stern L, Iqbal N, Seshadri P, et al. The effects of low-carbohydrate versus conventional weight loss diets in severely obese adults: one-year follow-up of a randomized trial. Ann Intern Med. 2004;140(10):778-85.

[6]Volek J, Sharman M, Gómez A, et al. Comparison of energy-restricted very low-carbohydrate and low-fat diets on weight loss and body composition in overweight men and women. Nutr Metab (Lond). 2004;1(1):13.

[7]Paoli, A., Bosco, G., Camporesi, E. M., & Mangar, D. (2015). Ketosis, ketogenic diet and food intake control: a complex relationship. Frontiers in psychology, 6, 27.

[8]Paoli, A., Rubini, A., Volek, J. S., & Grimaldi, K. A. (2013). Beyond weight loss: a review of the therapeutic uses of very-low-carbohydrate (ketogenic) diets. European journal of clinical nutrition, 67(8), 789.

[9]Sackner-Bernstein J, Kanter D, Kaul S (2015) Dietary Intervention for Overweight and Obese Adults: Comparison of Low-Carbohydrate and Low-Fat Diets. A Meta-Analysis. PLoS ONE 10(10): e0139817. https://doi.org/10.1371/journal.pone.0139817

[10]Gibson, A. A., Seimon, R. V., Lee, C. M., Ayre, J., Franklin, J., Markovic, T. P., & Sainsbury, A. (2015). Do ketogenic diets really suppress appetite? A systematic review and meta-analysis in obesity reviews, 16(1), 64-76.

[11]Diabetes & Metabolic Syndrome: Clinical Research & Reviews

[12]Feinman RD, Pogozelski WK, Astrup A, et al. Dietary carbohydrate restriction as the first approach in diabetes management: a critical review and evidence base. Nutrition. 2015;31(1):1-13.

[13]Veech, R. L. (2004). The therapeutic implications of ketone bodies: the effects of ketone bodies in pathological conditions: ketosis, ketogenic diet, redox states, insulin resistance, and mitochondrial metabolism, prostaglandins, leukotrienes, and essential fatty acids, 70(3), 309-319.

[14]Hall, K. D., & Guo, J. (2017). Obesity energetics: body weight regulation and the effects of diet composition. Gastroenterology, 152(7), 1718-1727.

[15]Archives of Internal Medicine. 2009 Nov 9; 169(20):1873-80. doi: 10.1001/archinternmed.2009.329. Long-term effects of a very low-carbohydrate diet and a low-fat diet on mood and cognitive function.

Disclaimer

The information contained in **"The Intermittent Fasting 16/8 Lifestyle & The Keto Lifestyle -2 In 1-"** and its components, means to serve as a comprehensive collection of strategies that the author of this book has done research about. Summaries, strategies, tips, and tricks are only recommendations by the author. Reading this book will not guarantee that one's results will exactly mirror the author's results.

The author of this book has made all reasonable efforts to provide current and accurate information for the readers. The author and its associates shall never be responsible for any unintentional errors or omissions found herein.

The material in the book may include information from third parties. Third party materials comprise of opinions expressed by their owners. As such, the author of this eBook does not assume responsibility or liability for any third party material or opinions.

The publication of third party material does not constitute the author's guarantee of any information, products, services, or opinions contained within third party materials. Use of third party materials does not guarantee that your results will mirror our results. Publication of such third party material is simply a recommendation and expression of the author's own opinions of that material.

Whether because of the progression of the Internet or the unforeseen changes in company policies and editorial submission guidelines, stated as fact as of this writing may become outdated or inapplicable later.

Made in the USA
San Bernardino, CA
22 February 2019